Cholinergic Urticaria: A Guide t

Written and published by B. Page

Copyright 2014 by B. Page

This book is a <u>CholinergicUrticaria.net</u> production.

Copyright and Disclaimer

Copyright

Legal Disclaimer

While the author has made every effort to ensure this book only contains factual and helpful information at the time of publication, the field of medicine is rapidly changing. The author is not a medical doctor, and he is writing this book as an individual who suffered with this condition—not as a medical expert.

Doctors and researchers still know very little about the exact mechanisms behind cholinergic urticaria. Therefore, the reader should not view this book as a final authority on this illness. Furthermore, while the author will discuss various treatments, remedies, symptoms, and strategies to beat this disease, individuals suffering with it should always consult a doctor before trying any treatment (or ceasing to use any treatments previously prescribed). Some medications or treatments could prove dangerous or fatal if used without proper medical oversight.

No warranty is offered, expressed or implied, to suggest the information in this book will be safe, accurate, or viable in all situations (or to all people). Furthermore, while the author firmly believes that the advice offered in this book may help individuals suffering with cholinergic urticaria, this book should not be construed as a claim, warranty, guarantee, or representation of success concerning any of the treatments or ideas covered. By reading or accessing this book, you agree not to hold the author or publishers liable for any damages or consequences that may arise from the use or misuse of the information given in this book.

Introduction: From the Author

I had my first experience with the horrendous condition known as "cholinergic urticaria" when I was 18 years old. Before that time, I had the luxury of enjoying excellent health. Aside from poison ivy, chicken pox, the common cold, and a few bouts of strep throat, I had no major health issues growing up. I didn't even have food allergies, seasonal allergies, or asthma as a kid (lucky me).

After I had my first hives attack, however, my life quickly went downhill. What started out as a slightly obnoxious, tingly itch, eventually progressed into a debilitating stinging sensation that would come to dominate my daily life.

Cholinergic urticaria slowly led me to a place of hopelessness. Despite multiple doctor visits and a myriad of "home remedies," nothing seemed to help my condition. The condition did go into a brief remission for a period of about 2-4 years (for reasons still unclear to me), but it soon made a drastic comeback.

I soon began to suffer from bouts of depression. My attitude of "I can beat this" slowly turned into an attitude of "I'll always be tormented by this." I found myself obsessed with this condition. I constantly tried to understand why I had it, how I developed it, and how I might cure it. I would scour the Internet daily in hopes of finding the one random article that could give me an answer.

As my hives worsened, I often found myself wishing I would simply die. I can distinctly remember many nights of crying myself to sleep, hoping that I would simply drift into death and never awake to the torment of hives again. Unfortunately, I'd often awake in the middle of the night with a severe hives attack!

I would often ask, "Why me? Why do I have this horrible condition? What did I ever do that was so bad that I deserved this?" I felt like I'd been robbed of my entire life, and at such a young age, too. I was miserable!

I also withdrew from nearly every activity I had once enjoyed, becoming an essential recluse in the process. Routine tasks such as shopping became difficult for me. I started scheduling my entire life around my hives—"just in case I had an attack."

What's worse—no one seemed to understand what I was going through. My family didn't seem to think my hives condition was significant. My wife, though extremely sympathetic and loving, had difficulty in consoling me many times due to her own frustrations about my condition. Most doctors also seemed puzzled about my condition and tried to mask the symptoms with drugs or antihistamines.

During this time, I also dropped out of college and quit my part-time job. I was majoring in accounting and had accumulated about 96 credit hours (out of a 124-credit bachelor's degree). I had no idea what I wanted to do with my life (I hated accounting, though I performed well in classes), and the unbearable attacks of hives left me feeling as if my career was already over. I didn't know what was happening to my body. "Perhaps I have cancer. Or maybe I'm dying." I thought.

I eventually started, to my knowledge, the first website dedicated to the condition: CholinergicUrticaria.net. There, I documented my thoughts and experiences with this disorder. I would bounce around hypothesis after hypothesis and idea after idea in an attempt to understand this condition and cure it. Other people also graciously posted their experiences with this condition, which made me feel a little less like a freak of nature.

After suffering with this condition on and off for around a decade or so, and trying nearly every remedy under the sun, I eventually found my cure (by God's grace). I say the word "cure" cautiously, though, because I'm not "cured" in the real sense of the word (meaning, the condition is gone for good). In fact, I can make my hives come back at any time. However, I also know how to make them go away and stay away—and this has worked for me now for about three years.

Today, cholinergic urticaria no longer dominates my life. I am active in a local church (something I wouldn't have even considered a few years ago). I shop, exercise and sweat, run my own business, and enjoy life. In other words, I have a life again. I no longer suffer from the debilitating mental and physical anguish of this rare hives disorder.

After many years of suffering with this condition, researching it extensively, and trying every personal experiment/remedy I could, I thought it was time to write a book about my journey.

In many ways, cholinergic urticaria was the worst thing that has ever happened to me. In other ways, it was the best thing that's ever happened to me.

In conclusion, I want to thank you very much for purchasing this book. I truly hope it helps give you information, motivation, and relief from your hives. May God bless you in your own struggles with this condition.

Why I Wrote This Book

First, let me state that I did _not_ write the book for the following reasons:

> **-I didn't write this book to get rich**. I never expect to see this book on a "best sellers list." I suspect very few people in the world have this condition, and of those, many probably won't bother buying this book (*cheapskates!*). I'd honestly be surprised if I sold as many as 200 copies over my entire lifetime (which would be a colossal failure by most selling standards).

> **-I didn't write this book to pretend I'm some guru**. There's a lot of information I don't know about cholinergic urticaria. I view myself as nothing more than a former sufferer trying to help other sufferers. I'm no medical

expert or researching whiz. I'm just a man who happened to cross paths with this unfortunate illness.

Now that I have that out of the way, what *are* the reasons I wrote this book?

-I wanted to give others hope. Let's face it: Life isn't worth living if you don't have hope. A preacher once said that the worst thing about hell is not the daily torment; it's the fact that there is no hope of anything ever getting better. After feeling a deep sense of hopelessness with my hives, I'd have to agree. Hopelessness stinks.

However, there is hope for you. If I can overcome my severe cholinergic urticaria, you probably can overcome yours, too. Hang on to any shred of hope you have. Things can and will get better in time. Even if my 'cure' doesn't work for you, there are still many ways to manage this condition. Treatments will improve over time—hang in there. I'll do everything I can in this book to help you.

-I wanted to help others "cure" or improve this condition. Having tried nearly every "remedy" known to man, I'm going to tell you what helped and what didn't help. I'll also go into detail about exactly how my "cure" came about, and I'll tell you how I keep my hives in remission today— no prescription medication needed. I'll include as much useful information as I can to help you. After all, we have this horrible condition in common. I'm on your side. I desperately want you to feel better and overcome your hives. I've been there, done that, and wrote a book about it (literally).

-I wanted people with this condition to have a book they can give to family or friends to help them understand the torture they go through on a daily basis. It can be difficult explaining this condition to others. If you allow them to read this book, perhaps they can come to a better

6

understanding of what you're facing. I hope they can learn how to provide better support and encouragement for you, and help you identify ways you may be able to improve your hives.

-I wanted to document all I know about this condition in a cohesive way. While I have a lot of useful information about this condition on my website, it is somewhat disorganized. As I mentioned before, it contains a myriad of hypotheses and ideas I once had, as well as posts of my various experiments and lamentations over the years. This could all be confusing to potential readers trying to piece it all together in a proper timeline, and it can be frustrating trying to navigate the website (especially if you have a slow Internet connection).

Therefore, I felt that I should collect all of my thoughts and put them down in book format so that it would be easier to read. This is especially true for those who aren't tech-savvy, or for those who have an extremely slow Internet connection (or simply want a digital copy or paperback to keep). While this book will contain some content from my website, I've also updated and added information and arranged it in an organized way. I want this book to be of value to you, the reader.

-I wanted to show my support for cholinergic urticaria. While many informative articles have been written online (some long before I came on the scene), there was not a website dedicated solely to this condition (to my knowledge). I started the first website, and I now want to write, to my knowledge, the first book dedicated solely to this topic. This is my small way of raising awareness while making my own small contribution to this disorder (and the community of people suffering with it).

What to Expect in this Book

First, this book is not a scientific thesis. If you're looking for a technical book with diagrams and scientific lingo, you'll probably be disappointed. I'll do my best to cover some of the prevailing theories and research, but I don't intend to get too technical or detailed in this area. I wrote this book for the average person, not the Ph.D. researcher.

Instead, I want this book to be a comprehensive guide to cholinergic urticaria for the average person. I plan to include basic information about the condition (symptoms, common treatments, etc.). I'll also share my complete story for any value it may provide. Finally, I'll have a "challenge" section at the end that I've designed to guide you on a path that I hope will lead to a better quality of life for you. It may or may not help you, but I know that it helped me.

Table of Contents

Chapter 1: My Cholinergic Urticaria Story

I was 18 years old when my cholinergic urticaria first appeared. I had actually just turned 18 years old about three months before my first hives attack. I can still remember my attack quite well: I had just gotten out of the shower, and it was wintertime (cold). I went into my room to get dressed, which consisted of a pair of jeans, a t-shirt, and a sweater.

I was in an energetic mood that day, and I was hopping around and acting silly. Suddenly, during my rush of excitement, I became hot. I started feeling this strange tingling sensation all over my upper body. It was something I had never felt before. It itched (really badly), but at the same time it had a prickly, stinging sensation.

I began thinking to myself, "What in the world is going on here?"

I started scratching myself, yet it didn't relieve the itch. That's the thing with cholinergic urticaria—you have to scratch, yet it provides no relief. The sensation got worse. The feeling spread throughout my entire upper body (chest, face, scalp, back, etc.). I was in complete torture. I didn't know what was going on. My face and chest became red (flushed); I was freaking out!

After calming down, the sensation finally quit. "What was that?" I thought to myself. Little did I know that it was just a taste of what would come to be a major change in my life: It was cholinergic urticaria rearing its ugly head.

I soon developed cholinergic urticaria reactions regularly after that day, and it seemed that any time I got hot, excited, nervous, etc., I would start breaking out in the same itchy/tingly sensation. It was bizarre because this condition literally came out of nowhere. It was mostly on my upper body, and my skin would usually become flushed (red) where I scratched, leaving the marks on my body for several minutes after the reaction ceased.

During a strong reaction, pinpoint hives would break out on my arms and chest for a few minutes, and then they would disappear within 15-30 minutes after I cooled off. However, this only happened after I'd had hives for a while (initially I only had itching, stinging, and flushing), and the pinpoint red dots (hives) did not always come out during an outbreak.

In addition, if I could somehow cool myself off quickly when I started to break out (by rubbing an ice cube on my body, going outside in the colder air, or jumping in a cool shower), then it would stop the reaction immediately. "Weird," I thought.

The reactions seemed to get worse over the next month. At that point, I would break out in a hives rash if I did anything that caused my body to heat up (laughing hard, exercise, getting embarrassed, doing physical work, jumping around too much, etc.) I thought I was going crazy!

My First Visit to the Doctor

Eventually, I broke down and told my mother (I was still living at home at the time) that I had to go to the doctor. I felt like a freak due to my odd symptoms. I prayed that there was a simple cure for what was happening to me. I was wrong.

I made an appointment with my primary care physician, and finally, the day of the doctor visit came. I was nervous, yet hoping that I could put an end to this painful and humiliating experience.

The doctor walked in. "Hello. How are you doing today?" he asked. "I'm pretty good (not really, but it's a standard reply). How are you?" I responded. I then proceeded to tell him of my problem: "I start breaking out in this really intense itch, and it is really uncomfortable and painful. It mostly happens when I get hot."

The doctor stood there a minute. Then the diagnosis came: "You know, I think your problem is dry skin," the doctor said.

11

Dry skin? I thought to myself, "How in the world does dry skin make you develop hives?" He continued to tell me a few lotions that I should try.

"But, this is really intense. It's as if I am breaking out in a rash or something. Are you sure it is just dry skin," I asked. "Yes," the doctor said.

I went to the store immediately after the visit and bought the lotion he recommended. I tried it for a few weeks. Nothing happened— my hives were still there. I became frustrated. I called and asked for a referral to a dermatologist. I thought that maybe they would know more about my problem.

The dermatologist I went to was a friendly, older man. I was optimistic that he would be able to fix my problem of breaking out in this intensely itchy rash. After all, dermatologists specialize in the skin.

It was very warm in his office (rare for a doctor's office/hospital), and I was actually having a hives reaction while he was talking to me. I pulled up my shirt. "Hmmm, I can definitely see some flushing in your skin," the doctor replied.

He asked if I had an infection of any kind. I told him no. He looked puzzled. He then explained that for some reason, my body was "stressed." He prescribed me some pills—Hydroxyzine—which is a strong anti-histamine.

I immediately thought to myself, "Yes! Finally, I have a pill that will cure me." Or so I thought. I took the Hydroxyzine right away, and I was excited that I could finally put this whole experience past me. It only took about 1-2 hours for it to kick in, and it knocked me out completely. Some antihistamines have a tendency to make you extremely drowsy, and I fell fast asleep (even though it was still in the afternoon).

For the first few days, I really thought the pills were working. I just felt better. I was tired for those few days, but I didn't care so long as it was going to cure my cholinergic urticaria. Unfortunately, after my body started to adjust to the Hydroxyzine after about a week, the drowsiness stopped. I also started having hives attacks again. Bummer.

I called the dermatologist and scheduled another appointment. I told him the medicine wasn't working and that I needed to come back again. By the way, I was unemployed but a full-time college student at this point. I didn't attend the next semester because my hives were bad. In addition, I really wasn't sure what I wanted to do with my life anyway.

I went back to the dermatologist, and this time he gave me a shot. I am not sure exactly what the exact chemical was, but I do know that it was a corticosteroid shot. Looking back, it was probably something such as Prednisone, Kenalog, or a similar corticosteroid.

"Maybe this will help," I thought to myself. The nurse administered the steroid shot on the side of my buttock. It stung, but I have never been the type to fear needles or shots. I went home, and for the next few days, nothing changed. I was still breaking out, and the steroid shot had no apparent effect.

At this point, I lost hope. I was tired of taking medications that didn't help. I don't most medicines manufactured these days, anyway. Many times, I think they are more dangerous than they are helpful in the end.

Moreover, since nothing was working, and the doctors seemed stumped, I decided to stop seeking medical advice. I also stopped taking my Hydroxyzine. I reasoned that it made no sense to keep taking a pill if it wasn't helping me.

For the next few months, things were rough, but I survived. I avoided heat as much as possible. I also tried various "home remedies." For example, I tried lotions, I tried making it more humid in the house, I tried taking showers less frequently, changing detergents, changing soap, etc. Nothing worked. It was torture. I would also carry around a squirt bottle of water, and when I became hot, I would spray myself to cool my body down. This helped me avoid a hives reaction.

By summer, I was still breaking out, but I had not given up complete hope. I would walk outside and immediately have a reaction when the hot sun heated my skin. I was still 18 years old at this point.

My Hives Went Away

One day, in the month of May or June, I decided I was going to go outside on a hot day and give my car a detailed cleaning. At first, it was complete torture, and my hives were breaking out. I was itchy, and it was intense.

Then, something happened that didn't happen for months before: a drop of sweat. That's right, sweat! In the months before, I simply couldn't sweat. If I tried, I would break out in hives before I would even sweat. The disorder just wouldn't let me get hot enough to sweat. Instead, I would itch instead of sweating. Yet, I finally felt a drop of sweat. It felt great.

The hives reaction soon stopped, and I was outside on a hot day working and sweating. It felt so great that I worked most of the daylight hours detailing it. Curious, I tried the same thing the following day.

At first, I got itchy and had a hives attack. Then it quit, and the "greenhouse effect" in my car made it so hot that I began to sweat again. I worked all day again. Finally, my hives quit coming out over the course of the next week, and they pretty much went into remission for a few years.

I'll just stop right here and say that I'm not sure why my hives went into remission. Perhaps it was a slow release corticosteroid

14

shot (such as Kenalog), and it knocked down my immune system to the point where it wasn't bothering me. Alternatively, perhaps it just spontaneously went into remission (this can sometimes happen with cholinergic urticaria). I'll never know.

My Hives Return

My hives remission wasn't permanent, however, and my hives soon returned with a vengeance. How did my hives come back? Well, very similar to the way before. It was winter, and I was now about 22-23 years old. My wife and I had moved out into our own one-bedroom apartment. I was working part-time at a major retail store (I hated it), and I was back in college working on my business degree. I wasn't too happy with my situation, and I didn't know what I wanted to do with my life.

My hives slowly began to return, but I ignored them at first. The symptoms came on much more gradually this time, until I eventually had a bad reaction at work that caught my attention. It was very uncomfortable and painful. Not only did my hives come back, but also something even worse was happening: I was having a rash come out on the back of my neck. It was a small rash (about the size of a penny), but it was itchy.

The rash soon got worse, and spread to the back of my legs, neck, and parts of my arm. It wasn't contagious (my wife never developed it), but it looked kind of like ringworm. In fact, I thought it was ringworm, but after a few unsuccessful attempts at treating it with cream, I realized it was just a common dermatitis rash.

The only thing the rash responded to was corticosteroid cream. However, the hives did not change. In fact, they worsened over the next year. What I soon noticed, however, is that my rashes cleared up when I cleaned up my diet. This discovery led to a lot of diet experimentation.

15

I began removing known food allergens (wheat, dairy, etc.), and my rashes and hives improved, but my hives wouldn't disappear completely. This was very frustrating. However, I kept experimenting with diet (with little success).

Eventually, my hives became very severe again, and I had almost given up on the idea of ever finding a "cure." I tried exercising, but my hives were far too intense. I also tried all of the previous diet experiments, and while they would help my hives, they never seemed to cure them completely.

This eventually led me to a new "hypothesis" that went a little something like this: Perhaps my hives were being caused by too much of an allergic response in my body. I knew that if I ate certain foods, my hives would skyrocket in intensity and rashes developed. On the other hand, I also knew that removing foods seemed to help my hives and it cleared my rashes.

Therefore, I formulated a new approach: I would try to eliminate anything that could cause an allergic response (food, environmental stuff, visceral fat, etc.). This led to new diet experimentations (and an allergy elimination diet), a new exercise regimen, and so forth (I'll discuss this in more detail in the "How I Cured My Cholinergic Urticaria" chapter).

After nearly eleven years of sporadically dealing with cholinergic urticaria, by the Grace of God I was able to overcome my hives. I've been able to manage my hives by eating a careful diet, continual exercise, and more.

In the remainder of this book, I'll discuss everything that worked for me, and I'll include a lot of basic information about cholinergic urticaria, too. Let's start with the basics in the next chapter: What is cholinergic urticaria, exactly?

Chapter 2: What Is Cholinergic Urticaria, Exactly?

Cholinergic urticaria is one of the physical urticaria subtypes, although some classify it as "other urticaria types." It is characterized by a hypersensitive response in the skin following an increase in body temperature, especially when the body's temperature increases enough to illicit a sweat response. To put it another way, cholinergic urticaria is a type of hives that erupts on the skin when a person suffering with the disorder experiences a sudden increase in body temperature.

What's interesting to note is that a person with cholinergic urticaria can experience a hives reaction with either passive or active heating of the body. Examples of active heating include any physical activity such as exercise (or physical activity), nervousness, or laughing. Examples of passive heating would include entering a hot building, taking a hot shower, standing in the sun, or entering a sauna.

Cholinergic Urticaria Etymology

Let's back up a moment and start at the very beginning: the name. Cholinergic urticaria gets its name from two sources:

> **-Cholinergic** - (pronounced "Cole-In-Urge-Ick") - This word means "related to acetylcholine." The first part of this word (choline) is derived from the Greek root *khole*, which means, "bile." Choline is an important part of acetylcholine, a common neurotransmitter.

> The second part of this word (ergic) comes from the Greek word *ergon*, which means, "work." Taken together, choline + ergic means, "related to acetylcholine," or, "works with acetylcholine." Acetylcholine is a chemical used in the parasympathic nervous system, and it seems to be involved in cholinergic urticaria reactions.

17

-Urticaria - (pronounced "Urr-Tick-Area") - This is a medical term for hives. The name comes from the Latin word *urtica*, which means, "nettle." A stinging nettle is the name of a plant that has small hair-like needles that create a stinging sensation in humans when touched.

During an urticaria (hives) reaction, mast cells break down and release histamine. This chemical produces a very prickly and itchy feeling in the skin, and it can lead to hives (small bumps), flushing (redness), and wheals (raised areas) on the skin's surface.

Cholinergic urticaria sufferers, for simplicity's sake, sometimes call the condition "heat hives" or "heat allergy." The term "prickly heat" is also used, although there is an actual condition called "miliaria rubra" that is more commonly referenced by that term.

In online forums, articles, or comments, people commonly abbreviate cholinergic urticaria as "CU," although this can be confusing since the same abbreviation is used for "chronic hives." Some people just refer to it as hives.

Cholinergic Urticaria Origins and History

Urticaria (general hives) is a condition that has plagued humanity for ages, probably even as early as the dawn of mankind. Even ancient medical documents mention the symptoms of general urticaria (and other similar skin rashes).

Hippocrates noted the symptoms of urticaria as early as the 4th century, associating it with "stinging nettles" and "insect bites."

(Source: Humphreys F. Major landmarks in the history of urticarial disorders. Int J Dermatol 1997; 36: 793-6).

The Yellow Emperor's Inner Classic, an ancient Chinese medical text, also describes urticaria as 'Feng Yin Zheng,' which means "wind-type concealed rash."

(Source: Rook A. The historical background. In: Warin RP, Champion RH. Urticaria. London: Saunders, 1974: 1-9).

Lastly, even the Bible references various skin diseases that plagued the Israelites. In the book of Leviticus, God gives Moses instructions for the priestly handling of these various skin rashes: "When a man shall have in the skin of his flesh a rising, a scab, or bright spot, and it be in the skin of his flesh like the plague of leprosy; then he shall be brought unto Aaron the priest, or unto one of his sons the priests." (Leviticus 13:2)

These ancient references reveal that urticaria is nothing new; it's been around a long time. However, this brings up an interesting question: How long has *cholinergic urticaria* been known, medically?

As medical knowledge advanced, urticaria began to be classified into different types, and it didn't take long for doctors and researchers to realize that some types of urticaria developed due to a physical stimulus.

As early as 1799, a doctor named Borsch mentioned solar urticaria by name (1). Frank mentioned cold urticaria, a type of hives very similar to cholinergic urticaria, in 1799 (2). The earliest known mentioned of cholinergic urticaria, however, wasn't until 1924 in JAMA by Duke (3).

(Source 1: Borsch JF. De purpura urticata, quam vocant "die Nesselsucht". Med Diss Halle, 1719.)
(Source 2: Frank JP. De curandis hominum morbis epitome. 1792; 3: 104 Mannheim.)
(Source 3: Duke WW. Urticaria caused specifically by the action of physical agents. J Am Med Ass 1924; 83: 3.)

From there, cholinergic urticaria is mentioned sporadically in medical literature. Even though it wasn't documented until 1924, individuals likely suffered with it long before that. Given the rampant misdiagnoses of this condition today, and the level of

19

general ignorance among general medical practitioners, it wouldn't surprise me if this type of hives has existed for centuries, if not a few millennia.

Cholinergic Urticaria Types and Subtypes

Researchers often try to divide cholinergic urticaria into different subtypes. These types are based on various studies and tests conducted by researchers. I should note that there is some disagreement among what subtypes exist, and there does not seem to be a consensus about these subtypes at this time. Nevertheless, I'll describe some of the commonly suggested subtypes below.

In a study by Nakamizo S, Egawa G, Miyachi Y, and Kabashima K., cholinergic urticaria was divided into four subtypes: Cholinergic urticaria with poral occlusion, acquired hypohidrosis, sweat allergy, and idiopathic.

(Source: Nakamizo S, Egawa G, Miyachi Y, Kabashima K. Cholinergic urticaria: pathogenesis-based categorization and its treatment options. J Eur Acad Dermatol Venereol. Jan 2012;26 (1):114-6)

An article published by Toshinori Bito, Yu Sawada, and Yoshiki Tokura suggested only three subtypes: Cholinergic urticaria with sweat hypersensitivity, anhidrosis or hypohidrosis, and idiopathic.

(Source: https://www.jstage.jst.go.jp/article/allergolint/61/4/61_12-RAI-0485/_article)

Poral occlusion is an interesting concept, primarily because other "poral occlusion" disorders such as miliaria rubra or tinea versicolor also exhibit symptoms similar to that of cholinergic urticaria. Some studies have found normal sweat gland functions in cholinergic urticaria sufferers, while others have suggested an abnormality or obstruction in the sweat gland functions of cholinergic urticaria.

For a long time, I suspected poral occlusion to be a cause of my own cholinergic urticaria; however, I no longer feel this is a cause for most people. Excess protein (keratin), bacteria or bacterial waste, fungus, and so forth most often cause poral occlusion. Nearly all of these things can be resolved with appropriate treatments. This is why I am somewhat skeptical of it being a major cause for most people with cholinergic urticaria. Nevertheless, it could be a cause in some people.

Hypohidrosis (reduced sweating functionality) affects many people with cholinergic urticaria, although I'd be hesitant to include it as a subtype of the disorder as the researchers did. With my own experience, I had years in which I could sweat normally, although I'd have to endure a minor reaction first. In addition, a non-scientific poll I asked on the cholinergicurticaria.net site revealed that 43.47% noticed a decrease in the ability to sweat, while 42.9% did not. Approximately 13.64% weren't sure.

Alternatively, I also had periods in which I couldn't sweat at all (anhidrosis), particularly when my hives were very severe. Therefore, hypohidrosis or anhidrosis seemed to be correlated with the severity of my symptoms, which fluctuated over time. Therefore, it doesn't seem like an actual subtype to me, but rather, it is more of an associated symptom. This may not be true for all cases, however.

Several studies have mentioned an allergy to sweat serum or even to the acetylcholine neurotransmitter. Fascinating experiments have also taken place whereby various researchers extracted sweat from a cholinergic urticaria patient and later injected it to see if it elicited a hypersensitive response. Some did exhibit this reaction, while others did not. I never had this test, and given the fact that my hives improve so much on my diet, it seems that I did not have a hypersensitivity to my sweat.

Idiopathic simply means that the cause is "unknown." In other words, the cholinergic urticaria didn't fit with the other subtypes, and they had no clue what was causing it. Therefore, they lumped into the "idiopathic" classification.

Again, there is still much to learn about cholinergic urticaria, and these subtypes aren't conclusive. They may change as time goes on, especially as researchers conduct more experiments and gather more information.

Duration

Unlike some disorders, cholinergic urticaria has no set duration. Individuals may suffer with it for weeks, months, years, or even decades before it goes away. In some cases, it may never go away (although treatments are available to reduce symptoms). In addition, cholinergic urticaria may go away and then reappear over time, and symptoms may fluctuate from minor to severe.

It is normal for people to suffer intermittently with it throughout their lives. Doctors classify any duration longer than six months as "chronic." Therefore, if you've had cholinergic urticaria for over six months, most doctors would consider you to have a chronic case. That may sound alarming, but it just means that you have a persistent case of hives.

My own hives lasted a total of about 11-12 years, although it did go away for a few years within that period. On the cholinergicurticaria.net forum, the longest mentioned duration was about 30 years. In a non-scientific poll on the cholinergicurticaria.net site, over 70% had it for more than one year, with 16.53% having it more than a decade.

According to a Medscape.com, one study reported that the average duration of cholinergic urticaria was 7.5 years, with a range of 3-16 years. However, later studies revealed that some had a much longer duration.

(Source: http://emedicine.medscape.com/article/1049978-clinical)

Epidemiology

Cholinergic urticaria affects both male and females. The condition seems to affect men more than women, but both genders suffer with it. Women may notice an increase in the level of their symptoms during menstruation or pregnancy, which may be due to natural hormone fluctuations.

Cholinergic urticaria is not dependent upon geographical location, as the condition has been reported in all major climates. On my website alone, I receive traffic from all habitable continents. Over the past year, the largest sources of traffic to my website came from the United States (65.39%), United Kingdom (9.02%), Canada (5.90%), Australia (3.26%), and India (1.98%). The rest of the visitors came from nearly every other geographic location. The stats above do not represent the proportion of sufferers per location, as not all locations have the same development and technology to access the web.

In a non-scientific poll on the cholinergicurticaria.net site, 21.49% lived in a mostly hot climate, 5.23% lived in a mostly cool climate, 72.73% lived in a moderate or mild climate, and 0.55% lived in "other."

As you might imagine from the geographic data above, cholinergic urticaria also affects all races/ethnicities. On the cholinergicurticaria.net forum, most major races or ethnicities (Caucasians, Asians, African Americans, etc.) have reported having cholinergic urticaria.

According to a non-scientific poll on cholinergicurticaria.net, 69.81% had fair skin (Caucasian), 18.87% had tan skin (Hispanic), 8.49% had dark skin (African American), and 2.83% reported "other."

Cholinergic urticaria may worsen during winter months as the humidity levels drop and sweating becomes infrequent. This drop can dry the skin, and make it difficult for it to acclimate to sudden increases in temperature. In another poll on the cholinergicurticaria.net site, 26.5% said the condition improves or disappears during hot weather, while 55.46% said that it remained year-round; 18.29% weren't sure whether the condition disappeared during warmer months.

Cholinergic urticaria seems to appear most commonly during the late teenage years. However, it can affect nearly any age group. On the cholinergicurticaria.net forum alone, individuals have reported having this condition since near birth. Others have reported having children as young as 20 months old with the condition. It can also affect older adults, and individuals as old as 60-70 years old have reported suffering with it.

In a non-scientific poll, 51.23% of people reported developing it between 1-20 years old, 26.7% developed it between 21-30 years old, 12.81% developed it between 31-40 years old, 6.27% developed it between 41-50 years old, 2.72% developed it at age 50+ years old, and 0.27% couldn't remember the age of onset.

Mortality/Life Span

I haven't seen any major studies on the mortality or life spans of individuals with cholinergic urticaria. Since the disorder often goes away on its own, it likely has little to no effect on life span. In fact, many people have suffered with it for decades with no other known issues.

The only possible effect cholinergic urticaria may have on life span is with the use of drugs that treat it. One study suggested that long-term use of some antihistamines might result in an increased risk of brain cancer. Other drugs used in the treatment of the disorder may also raise the risk for cancers and other diseases.

The disorder itself normally isn't fatal. However, in the rare cases of anaphylactic shock, it could be life threatening. This is why individuals with severe cases of this disorder must take precaution when exercising or engaging in physical activity.

Very rarely has this disorder been associated with terminal conditions such as cancer. In those rare cases, the cholinergic urticaria seemed to be caused by the malignancy, and it resolved when chemotherapy was administered.

One of the greatest concerns I used to have is that something was wrong with my body, and I thought that I might be dying. I'm still here so far, and many others who suffer with it are still around. While you should always get a good check-up from your doctor to rule out any other diseases, the fact is that you probably won't die from cholinergic urticaria. Instead, you may have to settle for something a little more boring (heart attack, being hit by a bus, cancer, etc.).

Treatments

There is no known "cure" for cholinergic urticaria in the traditional sense. In other words, you can't take a single pill and be done with it. However, there are many treatment options available. Individuals with minor cases may not need any treatments. Individuals with more severe cases may seek treatments including antihistamines, steroids, corticosteroids, diet modification, and more.

I'll discuss more about the specific treatments in the "Cholinergic Urticaria Treatments" chapter. I'll also discuss my own "cure" in a later chapter.

Causes

The exact cause of cholinergic urticaria is still unknown. Researchers have hypothesized that it could be a result of an allergy to one's sweat, an excess release or unbinding of acetylcholine, allergic causes, poral occlusion, and more.

Ultimately, the exact cause is unknown, but there are suggested subtypes as I've mentioned above. I'll talk more about causes in a later chapter.

Signs and Symptoms

The symptoms of cholinergic urticaria include a burning, stinging, itching, and/or prickling sensation on the body when it becomes warm—especially when the temperature increase is enough to elicit a sweat response. These symptoms normally cease once the body becomes cool or sweat is released.

Small, pinpoint hives may form and later disappear. Flushing, a reddening and warming of the skin, may also appear on the body. When not experiencing a reaction, individuals with cholinergic urticaria often have no signs or symptoms. In some cases, there may be a reduction or elimination of sweat (hypohidrosis or anhidrosis).

I'll discuss more about the signs and symptoms of cholinergic urticaria in a later chapter.

Frequently Asked Miscellaneous Questions

-What type of doctor should I see if I have this? Dermatologists specialize in the skin. They are the ones who will be most likely to be familiar with your condition. Allergists can also be helpful, particularly if you also plan to do allergy testing or allergy elimination diets. Most doctors do not "specialize" in this disorder, but some may work with urticaria patients more often than other doctors may.

Since the disorder is relatively rare, many healthcare practitioners are ignorant about it. This can lead to frustration on the part of the patient, as well as a feeling of being alone. Nevertheless, I recommend individuals to seek out a qualified doctor to confirm a diagnosis, discuss treatment options, and to rule out other diseases.

-Does it always itch? Itching is a very common symptom of this disorder; however, not all people with cholinergic urticaria may experience itching. Some may have flushing and hives. Others may have a burning sensation. Read more about the symptoms in the "Cholinergic Urticaria Signs and Symptoms" chapter.

-Can I have itching with no hives or redness? Yes, it is possible to have an itchy, prickly sensation. Hives do not always form, especially in minor cases. In my own case, hives did not appear immediately—itching, stinging, and minor flushing were my first symptoms. As my cholinergic urticaria symptoms worsened, I also noticed small, pinpoint hives forming. Eventually, these hives became much more impressive and noticeable.

-How long will I have this? No one can say for sure how long you may suffer with it. It can last months, years, or even decades. I had it for about 11 years, with a few years of remission within that period.

-How should I treat this condition? There are many treatment options available to help you manage symptoms, and I'd advise you try various ones under your doctor's approval. The biggest thing that helped me was my own regiment of diet, exercise, and a few other things (discussed in the "How I Cured My Cholinergic Urticaria" chapter).

At the end of this book, I'll offer my suggestions of what people suffering with this should try to reduce symptoms (so long as you have your doctor's approval to try it).

-This disorder is ruining my life—help! It can be very frustrating dealing with this disorder on a daily basis. It is perfectly normal to feel discouraged, unmotivated, and even depressed. However, there is hope for you. I often felt gloomy and frustrated, but now I have my life back. There are many ways to treat this condition, and I've done everything I can in this book to help you. Don't give up hope. I also have a chapter offering tips on staying positive and motivated.

-I have another urticaria type besides this one. Is this normal? Yes, it is not uncommon to have other allergic disorders occurring concurrently with cholinergic urticaria. In fact, some studies suggest that you have a higher risk of developing cholinergic urticaria if you have suffered with other allergies. Some individuals have both cholinergic and cold urticaria. Others may suffer with conditions such as rhinitis, eczema, food allergies, environmental allergies, and so forth.

-Alcohol seems to make my hives worse. Is this normal? Yes. Many individuals have reported that alcohol seems to make their hives worse the next day. This is probably due to the vasodilation effect, which increases blood flow near the skin's surface, which may allow the body to heat-up more quickly. Cholinergic urticaria suffers should strongly consider limiting alcoholic beverages for this reason.

Aspirin, Ibuprofen, and other NSAIDS may have a similar effect of making hives symptoms worse.

-How can I connect with others who suffer from this? If you'd like to connect with others who have this, visit cholinergicurticaria.net. This website has a forum section where you can post questions, leave comments on articles, and more. In addition, you can sign-up for a free email notification so you can keep up with the latest articles, posts, and comments.

Chapter 3: Cholinergic Urticaria Signs and Symptoms

The signs and symptoms of cholinergic urticaria, by itself, can range from insignificant to severe. People may have vivid outward signs (widespread hives or redness), while having very little inward symptoms (itching or stinging). Others may have almost no outward signs, yet their inward symptoms may be severe. Still others may feel both horrible inward symptoms and vivid outward signs. There is much variation in the severity of this condition.

In this chapter, I'll try to cover the range of signs and symptoms a person can expect to experience with this type of hives, and I'll also describe what a person with this disorder feels when a reaction occurs.

What Are the Cholinergic Urticaria Signs and Symptoms (When No Stimulus Is Present)?

Signs and symptoms will generally not appear in people suffering from cholinergic urticaria until they are exposed to some heat stimuli. In other words, they'll look and feel perfectly healthy (no hives or itching) when they aren't having a reaction.

In my own experience, the only symptom I would feel when I wasn't exposed to heat was an increased "awareness" or "consciousness" of my skin. This was a very subtle symptom, however. I'd compare this consciousness to wearing an uncomfortable sweater on your bare skin—every time I moved it just felt "icky."

This sensation didn't hurt or itch, but it didn't feel normal. Other than this heightened skin awareness, I considered myself perfectly content and healthy (so long as I wasn't being tormented by a dreadful hives attack).

Cholinergic Urticaria Signs (During a Hives Attack)

A "sign" usually refers to anything that another person can objectively identify, whereas a symptom is something that only you feel. An example of a sign of cholinergic urticaria is a collection of hives on the skin that appear when exposed to active or passive heating (anyone could see this). An example of a symptom would be severe stinging or itching (only you can feel this).

Listed below are some common signs that may appear during a cholinergic urticaria reaction. Not every sufferer will experience all of these signs, but any of the following can occur.

In a non-scientific poll on my website, 81.42% of sufferers said that they experienced itching, stinging, and small hives; 10.32% reported itching and tingling only (no hives); and 8.62% reported flushed skin or rash/hives only, with no stinging or itching.

-Flushing of the skin- Flushing is a common sign with cholinergic urticaria, and it may occur in localized or widespread areas. Flushing is the reddening of the skin as blood vessels leak fluid near the skins surface (similar to "blushing" when embarrassed). The flushed skin is often warm and more red than usual. It may itch, burn, or have no symptoms (other than visible redness). If scratched, a small wheal (raised line) may appear. This wheal, along with the flushing, usually disappears once the reaction subsides.

Flushing will most commonly appear in the area in which the hives appear or the itching occurs. For most people with cholinergic urticaria, this would be the stomach, back, face, neck, or arms. It may also appear on the legs, although it is more common for the upper body to experience the majority of the signs and symptoms.

Below is a picture of flushing that would appear on my skin during an attack:

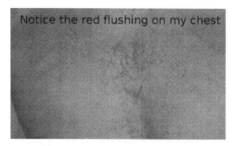

Notice the red flushing on my chest

-Small hives (urticaria) on the skin– People with cholinergic urticaria may see tiny pinpoint hives during or after a strong reaction. These hives are often small (about the size of a pen's point—about 1/16 of an inch), although they can be somewhat larger (about the size of a pencil's eraser—about ¼ of an inch). They are also usually red in appearance (sometimes with a slightly white center), although they may be flesh-colored.

In general, these hives only appear during or after a reaction. They often go away within 10-35 minutes, often leaving no trace. In rare cases, these hives may persist for up to 24 hours, but this is not the norm for most people.

Sometimes, these hives may have the appearance of raised goose bumps, maintaining a fleshly color with minimal redness. They may appear in an isolated, sporadic fashion, or they may appear in a widespread fashion. When my hives were most severe, it wouldn't be out of the question to see hundreds, if not thousands of them on my body. During one reaction, I was covered from head to toe.

Not all individuals with this condition will form visible hives; some people only experience flushing, itching, and a prickly sensation. My cholinergic urticaria started out with only flushing and stinging. Only after a few years did I begin to develop visible, widespread hives.

Here is a picture of the small hives that would appear on my skin (the photo is of the side of my stomach):

31

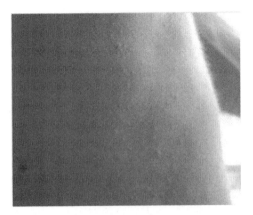

-Small wheals or raised welts on the skin– Small wheals (raised areas of the skin) may appear, particularly if a person scratches vigorously during an urticaria episode. These often disappear once the reaction subsides.

These wheals are usually very small and look like red scratch marks. They are a result of the skin's hypersensitive state and the histamine release during the reaction.

-General anhidrosis or reduced sweat functionality– Some individuals with this disorder will have significantly reduced sweat functionality. Many sufferers find it very difficult to sweat, even after strenuous exercise or exposure to hot, muggy weather. Rather than sweating, sufferers often experience a hives reaction first.

In some cases, sweating may occur after the individual remains in the heated or physical environment following the hives reaction. In other words, some people with cholinergic urticaria may have reduced sweat functionality, but may be able to sweat after enduring a hives reaction.

Some people use "sweat therapy" as a means to reduce the symptoms of cholinergic urticaria, although this may not be effective for all sufferers. In fact, it may be dangerous for those who suffer with anaphylactic shock. I'll discuss this in more detail in another chapter.

-Fainting- This is a rare sign of cholinergic urticaria, however, it has been reported in severe reactions.

-Increased Salivation- This is another rare sign of cholinergic urticaria, but there may be an increase in salivation (fluid production in the mouth) in some individuals after a severe reaction.

-Angioedema- Angioedema is the swelling of tissue under the skin. This is also rare, but some sufferers have reported swelling of the lips, eyes, face, and other body parts following a strong hives attack. Individuals at risk for this should ask their doctors about an EpiPen (an emergency injection used to calm severe swelling episodes).

-Anaphylactic Shock- While this is also rare, people with severe cholinergic urticaria have experienced anaphylactic shock. An allergic reaction happens rapidly in this very serious condition. The symptoms usually include difficulty breathing, change in blood pressure, and more. Individuals at risk for this should also ask their doctors about an EpiPen.

Cholinergic Urticaria Symptoms (During a Hives Attack)

-Uncomfortable skin sensation when warming- Individuals may feel a slightly uncomfortable feeling on the skin as their bodies increase in temperature. This is often an early indicator that a hives reaction is imminent. At this point, a rapid reduction in body temperature, or ceasing physical activity, may thwart the hives reaction.

-A prickly, tingling, or stinging sensation on the skin (which may feel slightly painful or uncomfortable) - This often occurs along with the itching. It often feels as if someone is pricking the individual with a small needle. This sensation can occur simultaneously over the entire body with the feeling of hundreds of "pricks" occurring in random places within seconds. They often sting and itch simultaneously.

This feeling often occurs slowly at first, with isolated pricks at the beginning of a hives reaction. As the reaction continues, the pricks may intensify in pain/itching and become widespread. This feeling often ceases when the heat stimulus is removed (or when the reaction subsides).

-Extreme itching (pruritus) during the hives reaction - This may occur anywhere on the body, but it commonly occurs on the face, scalp, and upper torso. Some individuals also feel the sensation on the legs. It may affect different parts of the body at different times.

The itching often occurs in waves and random points all over the body during the reaction. Individuals often feel compelled to scratch vigorously to soothe the itch; however, scratching does not resolve the itch. This extreme itching usually happens along with the "pricking" sensation above. It stings and itches so badly that you can't avoid scratching; however, scratching never quite soothes it.

People suffering with this condition may want to keep their fingernails short to avoid damaging the skin.

-Burning sensation on the skin– Individuals may feel as if their skin is burning during a reaction. For some, this is the primary symptom. For others, a burning sensation may occur as the reaction subsides and the "pricking" feeling stops. Other individuals may feel no burning sensation at all.

-Lethargy- A feeling of tiredness may develop after experiencing a cholinergic urticaria episode. This may be due to the large release of histamine, the energy used scratching, or the emotional effects of experiencing such intense stinging and itching.

A hives reaction may leave a person feeling so drained that they feel as if they must sleep or avoid strenuous activity for the remainder of the day.

-Headaches- A headache may also develop after experiencing a severe hives reaction.

-Abdominal Cramping- In severe cases, abdominal cramping may occur after a severe hives reaction. This is probably due to either the large histamine release or the effects of stress on the nervous system.

Quick Facts about Cholinergic Urticaria Signs and Symptoms

While the signs and symptoms of cholinergic urticaria can vary, here are a few simple facts to keep in mind:

> **-Symptoms may appear any age.** Cholinergic urticaria most commonly appears in the teenage years of life; however, very young children or elderly people have also reported having this condition.

> **-Symptoms may appear spontaneously.** A person may be perfectly fine one day and suddenly develop this condition the next day. This condition can also disappear spontaneously in the same fashion. Alternatively, symptoms may also appear or disappear gradually.

> **-Symptoms may first appear (or worsen) during winter months**. This is probably because sweating is infrequent, humidity levels are far lower, and the body must attempt to acclimate to sharp differences in temperature.

> **-Not all people with cholinergic urticaria will form tiny hives**; some may only feel intense itching, stinging, burning, or redness.

> **-Not all people with cholinergic urticaria will feel stinging and itching.** Some may have only visible symptoms such as hives or redness. I used to refer to these

people as the "blessed ones," as the physical pain and itching was by far the worst part of this disorder for me.

-Cholinergic urticaria reactions can occur suddenly when exposed to heat or emotional stimuli. Reactions may also appear gradually. Symptoms may appear differently based on the severity of the person's condition, as well as the temperature difference (large temperature differences may evoke stronger reactions).

-Individuals with severe cases of this disorder may have multiple reactions per day, each with equal severity. When my hives were worst, I would experience as many as 5-10 reactions per day, exploding each time in a new batch of hives, itching, and redness.

-Individuals with light to moderate cholinergic urticaria may only have one significant reaction per day, as the reaction may deplete their histamine levels and allow for a minor break from symptoms for a few hours.

-Signs and symptoms of cholinergic urticaria may evolve or change over time. For example, my symptoms primarily started out with little more than flushing and a frustrating stinging/itching sensation. However, over time small hives would develop in a very dramatic fashion, along with even more intense itching, stinging, redness, and lethargy. At some points, my hives were only mild, while at other times my hives were severe.

-Symptoms usually develop due to a systemic increase in temperature, not a localized increase. For example, if I placed a heating pad on my stomach, it usually wouldn't cause a reaction—even though the heating pad was very hot. However, if the heating pad caused my overall body temperature to increase after a few minutes, I would have a reaction. This may be due to the fact that a systemic increase in temperature activates the hypothalamus to send signals through the body to sweat, which then leads to the reaction.

-Symptoms may occur concurrently with other allergic or urticaria disorders. For example, a person may have both cholinergic urticaria and cold urticaria. Allergic disorders such as asthma, eczema, food allergies, and other similar conditions may also occur alongside cholinergic urticaria. I'd often develop slight eczema rashes and food sensitivities along with my hives condition.

How Cholinergic Urticaria Reactions Progress

How does a cholinergic urticaria reaction progress? What does a person feel as this condition begins to occur? That's a great question. While this may vary, I'll do my best to explain what I felt in my own words. However, I must admit that words alone can never accurately describe the feeling of agony that overwhelms a person as they feel the intense pricking, stinging, and itching.

First, I'll briefly outline what a person with cholinergic urticaria goes through in short, list format. Then I'll describe it in more detail.

> **-A person experiences some stimulus to make their systemic body temperature increase** enough to evoke a reaction (exercise, spicy foods, laughter, hot weather, etc.)

> **-A person then quickly feels an uncomfortable sensation**, similar to a "tightening" or "heightened awareness" of the skin.

> **-A person then typically feels isolated "pricks" on the skin**, which sting and itch in an indescribable way.

37

-**The stinging and itching may then quickly spread** over the entire body, or just an isolated area (such as the upper torso).

-**The person may begin scratching frantically** to soothe the sensation that is erupting all over the body, but the scratching rarely soothes the pain and itching.

-**Visible signs may begin to appear as this reaction spreads**, or the visible signs may not appear for a few minutes later. These signs can include small hives, flushing, wheals, etc.

-**The stinging, burning, and/or itching sensation may begin to subside** after the intense reaction. This is especially true if the body becomes cool, releases sweat, or depletes the histamine levels. In severe cases, the reaction may not cease unless the body becomes cool.

-**The hives, redness, wheals, or other physical symptoms may begin to dissipate** within mere minutes, usually leaving no trace of their appearance. Only rarely do these visible signs persist for hours.

-**The person may then feel tired or frustrated**. They may also have depressing thoughts.

-**The reaction has ended**, the visible symptoms have resolved, and the person finally feels normal again.

-**All of the above can happen within 15 minutes**. The initial reaction can appear within seconds. The reaction may persist for several minutes, and the hives usually clear up within 10-15 minutes after the reaction ceases.

Now that I've described what a reaction is like in the above format, I'll go into a little more detail.

For me to experience a cholinergic urticaria reaction, I'd have some stimulus to evoke the reaction. This could be anything that increased my systemic body temperature: Exercise, eating something spicy or acidic, laughing hard at a joke, physical intimacy, getting excited, or going from 20 degrees outdoors into a building with the thermostat set on 80 degrees.

When that happened, I'd often feel my skin becoming more and more uncomfortable as I'd feel my body becoming warmer. This would often worry me because I'd know a reaction was imminent. If I could cool down rapidly, then the reaction would cease, and I'd be fine. If the heat stimulus continued, however, the reaction would quickly progress to the next step.

The next step would be a few random "pricks" on my skin, followed by a strong urge to scratch it to relieve the sting/itch. This feeling was unlike anything I'd ever felt before. If I were to try to illustrate it, I suppose I could say it feels similar to the sting of an ant, mosquito, or perhaps a sweat bee. It was a very fine "prick," but it was enough to get my attention and make me immediately want to scratch at the area.

Let me put it another way: If the government could find a way to make this reaction occur scientifically, it would be an amazing torture device to use against terrorists or spies. I guarantee that even the most stubborn spy or terrorist would start talking if you tortured them with a severe bout of cholinergic urticaria!

This pricking, stinging, and itching sensation would slowly occur more rapidly, and it would cover more areas of my body. It may have started as a couple of isolated pricks/stings on my forehead, chest, or back, but it would quickly progress to a widespread sensation of agony. I'd also begin turning a little red on my chest or face (flushing).

I'd like to stop right here and point out that, even at this point, I'd be able to stop the reaction if I could quickly cool my body; and in my desperation to avoid an attack, I often did so. I've used about every trick you can imagine to cool myself down. I've used ice cubes on my body; I've kept squirt bottles filled with water in the refrigerator to cool myself off; I've jumped in cold showers; I've ran outside into 20 degree weather with my shirt off; I'd stand in front of the freezers at Walmart while shopping—the list goes on and on.

Assuming that I didn't stop the reaction by one of the desperate measures above, this reaction would persist for a few minutes. Small, red hives would then often form on my body, especially when my hives were more severe. Raised scratch marks (wheals) would also appear, and my skin would often be red and blotchy. These visible signs would usually be concentrated on my upper torso/arms/face, but they would also sometimes extend down into my legs.

While all of this was happening, I'd be scratching myself all over in a frantic attempt to stop the pain and itching. If it was in the privacy of my own home, I didn't mind. If it was in public, however, I'd feel so embarrassed. I'd do my best to "mask" my scratching by doing it as seldom as I could. I'd excuse myself to the restroom or rush out to the car, and then I'd have a scratch-a-thon. I'd move my hands as quickly as I could while scratching all over my scalp, back, stomach, arms, face, etc.

It would often be so frustrating; I just wanted to peel my skin off. It would feel as if it was stinging right below the surface, and if I could just peel it back, perhaps I could ease the sensation. It was horrible.

As the reaction would slowly subside, I'd finally start to feel a sense of relief. Any visible signs—the hives, wheals, or flushing—

would start to diminish within 10-15 minutes. After that, I'd look fine. I'd often be exhausted, but I'd look as if nothing had happened.

All of this would take a severe toll on me. It would drain me going through a reaction—emotionally, mentally, and physically. Sometimes, having just one reaction was enough to put me in a depressed mood for the rest of the day. I'd often ask, "Why me?" Life seemed so unfair. I felt as if I'd never find a cure, and I'd have no life.

I'd also develop a headache many times, particularly after a severe attack of hives. Of course, I couldn't sweat most days, either. Early on, I usually could sweat after enduring some itching. This was when my hives were only moderate. In my final years of suffering with this, however, I couldn't get sweat out at all—ever! I probably went an entire year or two without sweating.

As I've stated in this chapter, not everyone will experience the same symptoms. Some may have almost no stinging/itching but will experience visible hives. Some may have only minimal discomfort, whereas some will feel an almost unbearable sensation.

However, the signs and symptoms I described in my own words above affected me on a regular basis. That's what I felt when I had a reaction (for over a decade)—and it wasn't fun!

41

Chapter 4: Cholinergic Urticaria Causes/Triggers

What causes cholinergic urticaria? That's a tricky question because people may mean different things when they ask that. First, people may mean, "What causes (or triggers) the symptoms of cholinergic urticaria?" That's an easy question to answer. However, that's not what most people want to know. What most people want to know is, "What causes the condition to develop in the first place?" That's really the BIG question, and it isn't so easy to answer.

I'll start with the easy question (hey, I'm lazy).

What are the Triggers that Cause Cholinergic Urticaria Symptoms to Appear?

Cholinergic urticaria symptoms develop in response to an increase in body temperature, especially one that would cause a sweat response. This increase in body temperature must be systemic.

In other words, heating an isolated part of the body normally won't cause a reaction in most sufferers (unless it eventually causes the whole body to become warm), but an overall increase in body temperature would. In fact, I could often lay a hot heating pad on my stomach, yet I wouldn't develop a reaction because my systemic body temperature didn't increase.

The heat stimuli can be active or passive. An example of active heating would be exercise, whereas an example of passive heating would be entering a hot room.

Any number of activities, as you may imagine, can cause a cholinergic urticaria reaction. Some examples include the following:

Active Heat Triggers

-Any form of exercise (weightlifting, running, jogging, hiking, walking, etc.)
-Sports (football, basketball, baseball, wrestling, etc.)
-Sexual intimacy
-Exhibiting strong emotions that raise the body temperature (anger, laughing hysterically, embarrassment, frustration, excitement, shock, etc.)

Passive Heat Triggers

-Eating spicy foods
-Entering a hot building or sauna (or keeping the temperature too high in a room)
-Taking a hot shower (or sitting in a hot tub)
-Hot weather
-Sun exposure or tanning beds

What Happens (Physiologically) During a Reaction?

Now that I've covered the basic triggers of cholinergic urticaria, what exactly happens inside the body during all of this? I'll try to describe, to the best of my own ability and understanding, the basics of what happens in the body during a reaction.

I won't get too technical in this section. Even if I did, most people wouldn't understand it anyway (and I'm not sure if I totally understand it all, either).

The physiological process of cholinergic urticaria seems to be this (simplified format): Hypothalamus–>Acetylcholine–>Mast Cells–>Histamine Release–>Hives, Wheals, Itching, Stinging, and Flushing.

The Hypothalamus

The hypothalamus is a portion of the brain that contains a number of small nuclei with a variety of functions. Some functions include regulating body temperature, hunger, thirst, fatigue, and more. The hypothalamus is directly responsible for actively monitoring our body temperature. This is analogous to a thermostat being responsible for an air conditioning unit. It controls and monitors the temperature.

The hypothalamus is very much like a thermostat for the human body. When we get cool, our hypothalamus sends a signal to shiver, which makes us warmer by using energy. When we get hot, our "thermostat" (hypothalamus) sends a signal to our body to cool down. Our bodies "cool down" by releasing sweat from tiny glands located throughout the skin.

When our bodies release sweat, it produces a cooling effect by allowing evaporation on the skin's surface. The hypothalamus strives to maintain a consistent internal body temperature (a process known as homeostasis), which is typically around 98.6 degrees Fahrenheit. When our hypothalamus senses an increase in body temperature, it sends a signal to other receptors, which ultimately initiate a sweat response.

Acetylcholine

When our hypothalamus senses the increase in temperature, it sends an impulse down our neurons to activate the sweat glands. These impulse signals travel down through a network of neurons located throughout our bodies.

When this signal reaches the end of each neuron in the network, a neurotransmitter (acetylcholine) is released, which causes the next neuron to transmit the signal. For reasons currently unknown, this release of acetylcholine near the skin causes mast cells to degranulate.

Why does this happen? Perhaps the binding causes a change in surrounding proteins, which the immune system identifies as an "enemy." Alternatively, perhaps acetylcholine is released in excessive amounts. At this point, it is unclear exactly what happens in this phase.

Mast Cells

A mast cell (or mastocyte) is a resident cell of several types of tissues. Mast cells are a part of the immune system, and they contain many granules rich in histamine and heparin.

These mast cells are deposited in most tissues in our body, such as the skin, lungs, stomach, sexual organs, and so forth. When our hypothalamus sends a signal down our nervous system to sweat, acetylcholine, the chemical neurotransmitter, somehow causes surrounding mast cells to degranulate. When this happens, mast cells release the chemical known as "histamine."

Histamine Release

Histamine is a chemical created and stored by mast cells. Histamine increases the permeability of the capillaries to white blood cells and other proteins so that they can engage foreign invaders in the affected tissues. When our mast cells degranulate, the histamine inside of the granules is released.

This histamine release leads to immediate allergic symptoms: flushed skin (increased warmth/redness), extreme itching, small hives, and a stinging "prickly" feeling. This chemical is what leads to the very uncomfortable prickly and itchy feeling during a cholinergic urticaria reaction.

In summary, this is what generally happens to individuals with cholinergic urticaria during a hives attack:

-The brain's hypothalamus region detects an increase in body temperature.

-The hypothalamus then sends a signal down a neuron chain to activate the sweat glands
-These neurons release the neurotransmitter "acetylcholine."
-Acetylcholine, for reasons currently unknown, seems to cause a degranulation of mast cells in the surrounding skin.
-This rapid degranulation leads to a widespread histamine release in the skin's tissue near the sweat gland region.
-The release of histamine activates an inflammatory response in nearby tissue almost instantly, creating a very uncomfortable itching/stinging sensation, along with flushing and small hives.

The attack can usually be aborted if the individual rapidly cools down the body, which stops the signals from being sent to activate the sweat glands. If the body is cooled off manually, then there is no need for the hypothalamus to initiate sweat.

Strangely, once the body actually begins to sweat (which is difficult for most individuals with cholinergic urticaria), this reaction usually ceases. However, individuals are not always able to "sweat it out" and pass this phase of hypersensitivity.

What Causes Cholinergic Urticaria to Develop in the First Place?

In the previous section, I explained what triggers a cholinergic urticaria reaction, as well as some of the basic physiological mechanisms behind an attack. However, one question remains: "What causes cholinergic urticaria to develop in the first place?"

Unfortunately, this is the one million-dollar question, and it's hard to answer it with any certainty. Why is it that some individuals are healthy one day, and then the next day they develop this hives disorder that can last months or years? Why can the condition sporadically go away and then return? Why does diet seem to cure *my* condition?

These questions remain unanswered at this time. Doctors and researchers often consider the cause of cholinergic urticaria to be "idiopathic," meaning that the exact cause is unknown (or, as I like to say, it means they're idiots!).

Doctors and researchers also tend to divide cholinergic urticaria into subtypes, but this does little to explain why it develops. One of the suggested "subtypes" of cholinergic urticaria is due to an allergy to one's sweat serum. However, even if that is true in some cases, it still doesn't explain why the body suddenly identified the sweat as an allergen. I suppose you could argue that cholinergic urticaria develops in a similar way as other random allergies— perhaps it's a malfunction of the immune system.

Some articles have suggested the possibility of a defect in the nerve-sweat gland junction, meaning there is some abnormality here that leads to the reaction. However, the defect wouldn't seem to be genetic since the condition often goes away. Furthermore, in at least one study, the sweat glands of cholinergic urticaria sufferers were normal.

An article published by Toshinori Bito, Yu Sawada, and Yoshiki Tokura hypothesized that in individuals without cholinergic urticaria, acetylcholine is completely trapped by eccrine glands (causing sweat). However, in individuals with cholinergic urticaria, acetylcholine is not fully trapped and subsequently overflows to adjacent mast cells, evoking a reaction. Even though this article is very interesting, it still doesn't account for why this may begin to happen in individuals with cholinergic urticaria.

(Source: https://www.jstage.jst.go.jp/article/allergolint/61/4/61_12-RAI-0485/_article)

In summary, the exact cause of the development of cholinergic urticaria is unknown. We still know too little about it to say for certain, and even doctors and researchers seem stumped as to its etiology. However, there are a few cases in which an associated disease or allergy was suspected to initiate the disorder.

Cholinergic Urticaria Presenting as a Symptom of Underlying Diseases

While the exact cause of cholinergic urticaria is unknown, there have been isolated reports of cholinergic urticaria presenting as a symptom of another underlying allergic disorder or terminal disease. These reports are rare, and most individuals with cholinergic urticaria do not seem to suffer with the same disorders mentioned below. However, I'm listing them here because it is interesting to consider how or why these cases may have initiated cholinergic urticaria.

In one documented case, a link between copper/metal sensitivity and cholinergic urticaria was found. A person developed cholinergic urticaria symptoms due to a hypersensitive reaction to a copper IUD (birth control device) and copper dental fillings.

(Source: Shelley, W.B. et.al. "Cholinergic Urticaria: Acetycholine-receptor-dependent immediate hypersensitivity reaction to copper." *The Lancet*, April 16, 1983, pp. 843-846).

In another case, a female suffered with cholinergic urticaria for several years. Upon examination of her bone marrow, doctors discovered that she had hairy cell leukemia. After treatment with chemotherapy, the hives subsided.

(Source: http://www.ncbi.nlm.nih.gov/pubmed/10076710)

Many years ago, I also found a blog of a man who had developed cholinergic urticaria from the chemotherapy. He had some type of cancer, and after his first few treatments with chemo, he developed heat hives. I never could find his blog again, despite spending several hours entering search terms. It appears he must have deleted the blog.

The reports above should not alarm you; they are very rare and do not represent the normal individual with cholinergic urticaria. I just wanted to present them to show how cholinergic urticaria may be associated with other disorders or diseases.

Aside from these rare associations of cholinergic urticaria above, individuals on the cholinergicurticaria.net forum have also mentioned their ideas about what caused their hives.

A couple of individuals have suggested that their hives were caused by a vitamin D deficiency, which supplementation seemed to help. However, many have tried supplementing (me included) with no relief. Another individual reported that abnormal thyroid or hormone levels caused their cholinergic urticaria, but again, this hasn't been true for most people suffering with this disorder.

My Past "Theories" of What Causes Cholinergic Urticaria

I've had my share of "theories" of what causes cholinergic urticaria through the years. Most of these turned out wrong, and I no longer believe in most of them. However, I'll include a few of them below as a reference:

-**Hormonal imbalance**: I've often thought that there could be a problem with hormone production or secretion. This may lead to a complex biological problem in which the body becomes sensitive to sweating. This hormone imbalance could be the result of diet, stress, lack of vitamins, lack of sun exposure, undetected tumors, or other reasons.

One or two people did report on the cholinergic urticaria forum that their hives did improve upon thyroid or other hormonal treatment. However, many others have reported no benefit, and their hormone levels have tested within appropriate ranges. Therefore, this does not seem to be a mainstream cause for cholinergic urticaria, although it may be worth checking if you've had a history of thyroid or hormone issues.

-**Vitamin deficiency**: I strongly suspected that vitamin deficiency (especially vitamin D) was a cause of cholinergic urticaria. I researched heavily into how the majority of people are vitamin D deficient. Vitamin D plays a large role in the regulation of genes, some of which may be responsible for allergy or immune responses. In addition, at least one or two people have reported a remission of symptoms after from supplementing with vitamin D.

However, after my experimentation and supplementation, as well as other reports of people trying vitamin D with little success, I no longer feel that this is the cause for the majority of people with cholinergic urticaria.

-Autoimmunity: I've also speculated that cholinergic urticaria may be a type of acquired "autoimmunity," in which the body is becoming sensitive to its own natural chemicals (sweat or acetylcholine). This may be in conjunction with an autoimmune disorder (such as lupus), or it may be an autoimmune condition itself, which some studies seem to affirm with sweat sensitivity evidence.

However, this still leaves much unanswered, and it doesn't exactly help us understand what caused the body to develop an autoimmunity to sweat or acetylcholine. In addition, there is no causal link between lupus and other autoimmune diseases in relation to cholinergic urticaria (for the majority of sufferers).

-Fungal infection: At one point, I convinced myself that I must have tinea versicolor, a fungus that grows on the skin. Tinea versicolor can cause pigment discoloration in the skin, as well as blockage to sweat pores. This can result in symptoms similar to that of cholinergic urticaria.

I noticed slight pigmentation changes on my shoulder one day, and in my sheer desperation, I convinced myself that I must have this fungus. One of the treatments for tinea versicolor is to cover the body with a selenium sulfide solution, which I did using "Selsun Blue" shampoo.

Of course, I soon realized I didn't have tinea versicolor, and it didn't work at all to help my cholinergic urticaria. However, it did make me resemble the incredible hulk (I was a greenish-blue color!).

-Genetic susceptibility: I also speculated that cholinergic urticaria could be due to some genetic trait. However, no one in my own family has ever had it. A few people on the forum have mentioned a parent or family member suffering, but these cases seem rare. A few medical articles have mentioned a familial form of this disorder, but also expressed that it was extremely rare.

-Sweat gland obstruction: For a long time, I suspected that cholinergic urticaria was nothing more than an obstruction of the sweat glands, which caused acetylcholine to spill out and cause mast cells to break down. Some research articles even consider poral occlusion to be a subtype of cholinergic urticaria.

Reading about miliaria rubra, tinea versicolor, keratosis pilaris, and other "sweat gland obstruction" disorders reinforced my ideas. I even found another research article that stated that artificial sweat gland obstruction caused prickling and itching of the skin as sweat was released.

However, I eventually gave up on this idea. I eliminated virtually all sources of it: I scrubbed my skin, had a course of antibiotics, antifungal medication, etc. Nothing improved my hives.

There was also a conflicting study of sweat glands in relation to cholinergic urticaria, and researchers found no such obstructions or abnormalities. Furthermore, since my diet is directly correlated with my symptoms, I no longer feel that sweat gland obstruction is a major factor in most people's cholinergic urticaria.

-Bacterial or H. pylori infection: At one time, I suspected that I had H. pylori, a bacterial infection of the stomach. This particular infection causes symptoms of gastritis, but it is also known to cause odd immune system problems.

Considering my own stomach issues, I suspected that perhaps my hives were caused this nasty bug. I even made an appointment with a local doctor for testing. However, the test results were negative.

In addition, I also considered that my hives might have been caused by a bacterial infection elsewhere. However, I've had a course of strong antibiotics, and it didn't have any effect on my hives. I no longer feel that bacterial infections are a widespread cause of cholinergic urticaria.

-**Spider bite**: About six months before I developed cholinergic urticaria, I developed what appeared to be a spider bite on my face. It turned into a noticeable scab and left a scar. I'm not sure if it was a spider bite or not, but if it was, I theorized that it may have triggered an immune response. I also wondered if some allergic response to a bug bite might cause sweat allergy in some people.

However, I no longer believe this to be a major cause of my cholinergic urticaria.

-**Tanning lotion**: About eight months before I first developed cholinergic urticaria, I went to a tanning bed with a few of my friends. I never go to tanning beds, but we were preparing for our "senior trip" after graduating high school. The idea was to get a slight tan so that we wouldn't get sunburnt at the beach.

While I was there, I put on some accelerating tanning cream before using the tanning bed. Afterward, my skin started burning like crazy and got bright red. It was an odd reaction, and I've often wondered if the cream and subsequent UV light created some immune response.

Alternatively, it could have been some of the first signs that cholinergic urticaria was developing. Ultimately, I'll never know, but I'll never put that cream on my skin again (or go to a tanning bed)!

-Strong deodorant: A few months before I developed cholinergic urticaria, I also tried a strong deodorant. In high school, I sometimes had the problem of constant sweat under my armpits. This didn't cause any problems—it's quite normal—but I wanted to eliminate it.

I found some "extra strength" deodorant online, and I ordered it. I applied it and it did work, but it caused a lot if itchiness under my arms. I often wondered if the extra strong deodorant caused some sensitivity in my skin to the sweating process.

However, this doesn't seem to be a big cause with most people. In addition, since my diet seems to be correlated with my hives, it may not have anything to do with it.

-Environmental allergies: I also suspected that some environmental allergy was causing this odd reaction. Perhaps an allergy to soaps, pets, pollen, or something else caused my cholinergic urticaria. Many others have also reported high allergic responses to pet dander, dust mites, and so forth.

While I think environmental allergies can add to cholinergic urticaria symptoms, they don't seem to be a main cause.

-Food allergies or intolerances: I've also long suspected that there may be an underlying (unknown) allergy or intolerance to something in the diet or environment, causing increase an increase in IgE production (or other immune responses).

Since diet plays such a large role in my own cholinergic urticaria, I suspect that this may be true (at least, in my case it may be true). The fact that my diet seems to be directly related to my symptoms tells me food is involved. This could be in one of two ways: First, food could be directly involved due to an allergic response from eating certain foods, which causes inflammatory immune cells to build-up in my body.

Alternatively, I suspect it is also possible that my body lacks a certain enzyme to break down a substance in certain foods. Because this chemical isn't properly digested, it accumulates in my body. An example of a disorder with a similar effect is known as "Fabry's disease." In that case, individuals lack an enzyme to break down certain fats, which accumulate in the body over time, causing many problems.

Conclusion

Frustratingly, I admit that I have no idea what causes cholinergic urticaria to develop—even after all of these years of my experiments, researching, and pondering. As I mentioned above, my diet seems to be the biggest factor in my hives. However, this may not be true for everyone, and I still don't understand all of the mechanisms behind my own hives.

I hope that one day we will know so much more about this disorder. For the time being, my biggest desire is to help people overcome their hives so that cholinergic urticaria is no longer a major factor in their lives.

Chapter 5: Cholinergic Urticaria Treatments

At this time, there is no known "cure" for cholinergic urticaria. I've cured mine in a sense, and I'm no longer plagued by the painful symptoms (at least, as long as I stay on my strict diet). However, there is no known medical "cure" for this disorder in the sense of taking a few pills and being done with it. That's the bad news.

The good news, however, is that there are many ways to treat this condition and reduce the symptoms. Some methods and medications can reduce the symptoms so much that cholinergic urticaria will be little more than a minor annoyance. For people with severe cholinergic urticaria, however, treatments may only take some of the sting out of it (but it may be just enough for you to keep your sanity).

This chapter will cover most of the mainstream treatments that doctors and sufferers use to treat this condition. First, let me give a quick disclaimer:

- Never, under any circumstances, take or stop taking a medication/treatment without consulting a qualified medical doctor or health professional. I'm not a doctor.

- The treatments in this chapter may not be appropriate or safe for all people, especially those who are nursing, on other medications, or with other medical conditions.

- These treatments could prove dangerous or fatal if you do not take them with the supervision and approval of a licensed physician.

In addition, I will not discuss my current "treatment/cure" in this chapter—I'll have an entire chapter devoted to that.

Treating or Controlling Cholinergic Urticaria (without Medication)

First, there are a few ways you can reduce symptoms or prevent attacks without medication, and it makes sense to list those first. Cholinergic urticaria sufferers can often manage their hives or reduce symptoms (or the risk of a hives attack) naturally by doing the following:

-Avoid situations that cause hives. This probably seems like a no-brainer, but if you can avoid a situation that you know will cause an attack, avoid it. This could be as simple as avoiding spicy or acidic foods in public, not laughing too hard, etc.

I would often do outdoor tasks (mowing the yard or washing the car) in the early hours of the day so that it wouldn't be so hot outside. I'd also take special care not to run or physically exert myself when I knew I was at risk for an attack.

-Cool down rapidly. If you do have an attack, you may be able to stop it completely by quickly cooling yourself down. As I said before, I'd often jump in a cool shower at home, use a squirt bottle with cold water, take an ice pack, take off layers of clothes, and so forth.

-Don't overdress. Wear appropriate clothing to help keep the body cool. Rather than wearing a large hoodie, consider wearing a zip-up jacket that you can easily take off. Wear thin jeans/pants during the winter, and shorts or thin capris during the summer.

Select fabrics that are thin and breathable, such as cotton. Also, consider the color of clothing: Dark colors absorb the sun's rays, while lighter colors reflect them. Therefore, dress in removable layers, in breathable fabrics, and in light-colored shades.

Moisture "wick" shirts may also help. I never purchased any moisture wick shirts. However, a few people have indicated that they can help prevent an attack. This may be due to the thin design of the fabric.

In addition, a lot of your body heat escapes through your feet and head. Therefore, it makes sense to avoid wearing thick socks or hats. This way, your body heat can escape more quickly, and you can avoid overheating.

-**Make diet changes**. Avoid spicy or acidic foods, or foods that upset the digestive system. A few examples include vinegar, citrus, peppers, sausages/pepperoni, sour candy, and sour or spicy foods.

It would be a very wise decision to keep a food diary to determine any reactions you may have to foods, such as a stomach upset, eczema, rashes, or increased urticaria sensitivities. Making an appointment with an allergist may help with this, especially if you can get a food allergy test performed.

Just keep in mind that these tests are not exhaustive, but they may help you identify issues you may have with common foods. For example, many people with cholinergic urticaria avoid alcohol, as drinking alcoholic beverages seems to worsen the condition.

Eating less food is also helpful for many, especially if the person is obese or overweight. I know that when I would eat less food, my hives were a little less reactive as opposed to when I ate large quantities of food. This also seems to be true for people with exercise-induced anaphylaxis.

Aside from the tips mentioned above, an allergy elimination diet is something that benefitted me immensely, and it may be wise to do that along with a food diary. Eliminating troublesome foods played the biggest factor in controlling my cholinergic urticaria. I'll talk more about diet and cholinergic urticaria in a separate chapter.

-**Avoid unnecessary supplements, drugs, or medication**. If you take an unnecessary supplements or medications, it may be wise to eliminate them (with a doctor's prior approval). Some medications can contain chemicals or allergens that can aggravate cholinergic urticaria. A few examples of such medications could be Aspirin or Ibuprofen, which tends to thin the blood. Those medications always seemed to make my hives much more reactive.

Other examples include protein powders/fitness supplements, various vitamin supplements, etc. Although I do take a daily multivitamin (Centrum) and probiotic, you do have to beware. I took Men's One-a-Day multivitamin for a few days, and it caused blisters to form on my ears due an allergic reaction. Therefore, if you take any unnecessary medications or supplements, make sure they aren't causing any reactions.

Finally, it should be common knowledge that recreational drugs aren't going to do your health any favors. If you're doing any recreational drugs whatsoever (alcohol, cocaine, pills, injections, pot, cigarettes), I'd recommend stopping them as soon as possible. If you've learned nothing else from cholinergic urticaria, you should have learned this one fact: Your health is a gift that can be taken away at any time. Therefore, take care to preserve what health you do have.

-Use exercise or sweat therapy. Some individuals with cholinergic urticaria use exercise or sweat therapy as a way to induce frequent and regular attacks, thus, limiting the severity of the attacks. The idea is to force a hives reaction, which may induce the body to sweat with more regularity. It also causes a release of histamine during the attack, which temporarily reduces the histamine levels in the body. This reduces the intensity of the urticaria reactions for a period of around 24-48 hours.

This approach works well for people with mild forms of cholinergic urticaria. However, those with the more severe forms may not be able to use this method (or may need to stop for health reasons).You can do this via exercise (cardio or strength training), or any way that may cause sweat—home saunas/steam rooms, etc.

There was one point in which I could sweat, and I'd feel remarkably better after "sweat therapy." However, when my hives were most severe, I'd exercise for long stretches wearing a ridiculous outfit to induce sweat, yet I'd still never get a drop of sweat out. Even with the thermostat turned up to 80 degrees with a sauna suit, a large jacket, and thick pants on, I'd still never be able to sweat.

In addition, individuals with a risk of exercise-induced anaphylaxis or anhidrosis should not attempt this method, as it may result in a fatal allergic reaction or heat stroke. Finally, you should always talk to your doctor before you begin an exercise program, especially if you have cholinergic urticaria.

I'll discuss much more about how I was able to exercise with cholinergic urticaria, and provide some sample exercise routines and samples in a later chapter.

-Use good skin care techniques. Keep your fingernails short so that you can avoid damaging your skin while scratching. Try to select a soap that's hypoallergenic (I use Dove's sensitive skin). Try to get hypoallergenic shampoo, lotion (I use Eucerin Calming Crème), and detergent (I use ALL Free Clear). Anti-itch lotion may also provide minor relief.

In addition, try to take brief, tepid showers. Apply lotion immediately afterward to retain moisture in the skin. Avoid scalding-hot, 35-minute showers. I also highly recommend using a shower filter. These help filter out chlorine and other similar chemicals. I have one made by Culligan, and it simply screws onto a standard showerhead (it costs about $15-20).

Finally, maintaining a comfortable humidity is also important so that your skin doesn't dry out. I've experimented with vaporizers and humidifiers. I found that using a humidifier was best (it consumes less electricity, and has more control settings). I use one by Crane, and I'd highly recommend it.

-Avoid environmental allergens. Given that many people with cholinergic urticaria have reported sensitivities to dust mites, I strongly recommend dust mite-proof bedding. I got mine in early 2011. I recommend you avoid vinyl, as this can stink terribly at first and may not be as safe as less gassy plastics. Get one that covers your upper mattress and pillows, and don't forget to wash your bed sheets weekly in a hypoallergenic detergent.

Try to avoid any of your known seasonal allergies as much as possible. I know this can be difficult, but do what you can to minimize exposure to your seasonal triggers such as pollen, etc.

Finally, I love animals to death, but I'd never live with one in the same house. My mother had five indoor dogs when I was growing up. They'd bring in all sorts of pollen, pet dander, dust mites, poison ivy, and whatever else they rolled around in outside. She had to clean constantly, and the house stayed quite dusty.

I know most people love pets, but if you can, it would probably be best to avoid getting indoor pets. However, if you do have a pet and keep it outside, please have the decency to make sure it has proper shelter/food, especially on cold nights.

-Pray. I must have prayed thousands of times over the course of a decade for my hives to go away, and thankfully, they have. There was once a time in my life (in my brief atheistic years) in which I would have scoffed at the idea of prayer, but after having come to faith in Christ, I realize that God does indeed answer prayers. It isn't always instantaneous. It isn't always in the way we want. It isn't always a "yes," but God does answer prayers.

While I'm not the type to force my religion onto others, I would encourage you to pray about your hives daily. Pray for God to heal you. Pray for Him to give you wisdom in how you can treat or "cure" your hives. I'd often pray for God to forgive my sins, to reveal Himself to me, and to help me grow in my understanding of Him. He's done that and so much more. I am truly blessed.

In addition to prayer, mental relaxation techniques may also help you cope with attacks or stress of living with the condition. However, it will not generally cause the reactions to cease. Nevertheless, keeping calm and relaxing during an attack may keep it from intensifying.

Treating or Controlling Cholinergic Urticaria (with Medication/Supplements)

While I'd urge everyone with this disorder to pursue the most healthy and natural treatments first, medications can be helpful. Doctors and sufferers have used many different drugs to treat this condition, and I'll do my best to cover these various treatments in this chapter.

It is important to note that when you try to treat cholinergic urticaria, it can be very difficult to know whether the treatment is working. Sometimes cholinergic urticaria can go through cycles where the hives are very reactive, followed by a period of the hives being much less reactive. This can lead to the misconception that a treatment is helping, when in reality, the hives are just going through a period of less reactivity (for whatever reason that might be).

In addition, while I haven't tried all of the medications/treatments listed below, I have tried many of them. I'll add my own experiences and thoughts where appropriate. You're more than welcome to consult with a doctor or perform your own research on the medicines below to form your own opinions.

Vitamins/Supplements

You can buy most vitamins and supplements in your local store without a prescription, but that doesn't mean you should load up on them without consulting a doctor. You can overdose on many vitamins (such as vitamin D3), and the Internet is filled with whackos telling people to take dangerously high doses of vitamins, which could prove fatal.

I've taken many vitamins and supplements through the years (with mixed results), and other sufferers have reported some benefit from taking various types.

Here is a list of vitamins and supplements that may provide some relief (although I am not advocating doing them all simultaneously):

-Multivitamins (Centrum) – I still take a multivitamin daily, and I'd recommend them. This is especially helpful since I eat a very restricted diet, and I may not get all of the calcium and other nutrients I need to meet my daily requirements. A multivitamin probably won't cure your hives, but it may help you maintain healthy vitamin levels.

-Vitamin D3 –A couple of people on the cholinergicurticaria.net site reported that taking vitamin D supplements either helped or cured them, whereas most have reported little to no benefit. Most of the population has low levels of vitamin D anyway, and it may be worthwhile to have a simple blood test performed to check for a deficiency.

I did take vitamin D3 supplements for about a year or two; however, I eventually cut it out because it didn't seem to help my hives. Most multivitamins have vitamin D3 already in them, and you only need about 500-1000 IU per day. If you have a severe deficiency, your doctor can usually give you a shot. You can overdose on vitamin D3, however, so only take the amount recommended by your doctor.

Source: (http://www.cholinergicurticaria.net/vitamin-d-deficiency-and-supplementation-for-cholinergic-urticaria/)

-Vitamin B – Some visitors to the cholinergicurticaria.net website have also reported that vitamin B complex (or vitamin B6/B12) helped provide some relief. It did not cure their hives, but did seem to make the symptoms more bearable.

I also took this and did not see a benefit. Again, I would just caution you to check with a doctor and take a safe dosage. Even though some of these vitamins may be water soluble, it can be very dangerous to take them in high doses.

(Source: http://www.cholinergicurticaria.net/vitamin-b-or-b6-for-cholinergic-urticaria/)

-Fish Oil Pills/Omega-3 Fatty Acids – Some people have reported that taking fish oil or omega-3 fatty acids have helped reduce their symptoms. Others have reported that it didn't help at all.

I did try some, eventually, but it didn't seem to help my hives. Some news reports have suggested that high intake of these fatty acids could lead to increased risk of some cancers.

Source: http://www.cholinergicurticaria.net/fish-oil-pills-omega-3-6-and-cholinergic-urticaria-hives/

-Vitamin C – Vitamin C is a common vitamin that many people take on a daily basis. It also acts as an antihistamine because it has the ability to reduce histamine levels in the body. I did take high doses of vitamin C for a couple of months, but I did not notice any benefit or reduction in symptoms.

Nevertheless, since so many people take this regularly for its immune system benefit, it may be something to keep in mind.

-Probiotics – Probiotics contain "good" bacteria that benefit the digestive system. The majority of your immune system is found in your intestines, which makes sense considering that most foreign objects will be entering via that route.

My experience with probiotics has been interesting. On one hand, they have helped me in many ways. On the other hand, they didn't cure my hives. In addition, I have to rotate different brands because my body seems to adapt to them after a month or two.

When I had horrible stomach cramps and digestive issues (gas, bloating, diarrhea, cramping), they did help tremendously. I have also found that they reduce inflammation in my own body, and there has been some articles hinting that they may reduce many allergies.

I first noticed that they helped because I would often develop tiny red bumps on my hands, elbows, and so forth. When I began taking these probiotics, these bumps gradually improved, even without diet modification. My digestive system also improved, and it seemed as if my hives improved as well.

I'd recommend people with cholinergic urticaria to consider them as a way to help reduce overall inflammation in the body, as these bacteria help keep your immune system in check. I've used many different brands of probiotics: Digestive Advantage, Culturelle, Align, Enzymatic Pearls, etc. The one that seems to work well for me is Digestive Advantage, but I do alternate and take different ones. Again, your experience may be different so if one doesn't work well, you may want to try another.

One thing I found interesting is that when you take a probiotic, you'll probably notice a change in your bowel movements immediately. It may change it from diarrhea to solid, or you may use the bathroom more often or less often.

Probiotics, by themselves, will not likely cure your hives. However, they may help calm them down some, and you may notice the benefit of improved digestion and reduced inflammation (allergies, rashes, eczema, etc.) in your body.

Antihistamines/Mast Cell Stabilizers

Antihistamines are agents/drugs that serve to inhibit or prevent the release of histamine in the body. Histamine is a chemical involved in allergic responses and other biological functions in the body. For example, during a cholinergic urticaria reaction, the body releases histamine. This is what causes the "itchy" or "prickly" feeling.

These drugs are probably the most common drugs used to treat hives, and people often have mixed results with them. They provide a lot of relief for some people, whereas others receive very little relief.

You can purchase many antihistamines in a local drug store, or online from just about any retailer. Over-the-counter antihistamines do not require a prescription. Some antihistamines are stronger and require a prescription, although this can vary depending on your country's laws.

Common Antihistamines Include the Following:

-Vistiril/Atarax (Hydroxyzine)--(usually prescription)
-Claritin (Loratadine)
-Zyrtec (Cetirizine)
-Alaway/Zaditor (Ketotifen)
-Clarinex (Desloratadine)
-Allegra (Fexofenadine)
-Xyzal (Levocitirizine Dihidrochloride)
- Qdall (Chlorpheniramine Maleate)
-Benadryl (Diphenhydramine)
-Periactin (Cyroheptadine)
-Pepcid (Famotidine) (H2 antihistamine)
-Zantac (Ranitidine) (H2 antihistamine)
-Many more (usually by prescription)

Possible Side Effects/Precautions

Antihistamines can cause side effects, including upset stomach, drowsiness, irritability, dry mouth, headache, decreased urination, change in bowel movements, etc. Long-term use may cause additional side effects, such as a slightly increased risk of gynecomastia ("male breasts"), cancer, and more. Gynecomastia is mostly related to long-term H2 antihistamine use.

Also, if you are pregnant (or may become pregnant), some antihistamines are not recommended. They may also interfere with other mediations. For a full list of side effects and precautions, talk to your doctor and/or read the medication warnings for each kind of antihistamine.

One thing that you should keep in mind is people react differently to antihistamines. One may work perfectly for you, while the same medication may do nothing for another person with heat hives. Some antihistamines may cause significant side effects, whereas others may work with little to no side effects. Therefore, you really just have to work with your doctor to see which ones work best for you.

In addition, antihistamines do have a habit of becoming less effective over time. This was certainly true for me. I'd become adapted to most antihistamines after a mere week or two, and they'd become almost useless after that. However, after avoiding them for a few weeks, they'd be effective again.

My Experience with Antihistamines

I would use antihistamines quite a bit, but I never got much relief from them. They only took a little of the pain away. The one that was most effective for me was Allegra (Fexofenadine). It did help some, but it soon lost its effectiveness.

Benadryl would put me to sleep; Zyrtec would give me a terrible headache and stomach pain; and Claritin did nothing. Hydroxyzine also made me very drowsy. However, you may have a different experience than I did with these antihistamines, so don't let my experience keep you from trying them (if your doctor suggests doing so).

One thing I discovered is that sometimes antihistamines can be used together in different combinations (H1 and H2). Some doctors have also combined antihistamines with a proton pump inhibitor (such as Prilosec) for better results. This can be serious medicating, so you should discuss this option with a doctor as a last resort.

I only combined different antihistamine types (H1 and H2) when my hives were severe and I needed to reduce the symptoms for some important occasion. I would take an H1 and H2 antihistamine: Allegra (H1) and Pepcid (H2).

I would take the Allegra first, wait two hours, and then take the Pepcid. I've done this less than ten times in a decade, and I'd certainly not do it as a daily treatment. However, it did provide much better relief than just a single antihistamine. Please don't try this without talking to your doctor about the possible risks.

Anabolic Steroids

Anabolic steroids (muscle-building steroids) have also been used to treat cholinergic urticaria. In most instances, these steroids are reserved for severe cases. Individuals treated with anabolic steroids often have mixed results, and some articles have reported a reduction of symptoms with this treatment, while others experienced only temporary relief or almost no relief.

When treating cholinergic urticaria, the most commonly prescribed anabolic steroid is Danazol. Several online medical publications have published articles related to the experimental treatment of cholinergic urticaria with Danazol, an androgen steroid. Here is one sample of a source that studied the treatment of Danazol on cholinergic urticaria: http://www.ncbi.nlm.nih.gov/pubmed/16865874

The article suggests that Danazol was effective in reducing cholinergic urticaria symptoms. Other articles, however, have revealed that it is ineffective in some people, and some who previously responded well eventually experienced a relapse of symptoms.

Steroids are very serious drugs. You should only use them if your doctor prescribes them. According to most research articles, steroids were only used in extreme circumstances. They may provide some relief, but each individual should weigh the potential long-term effects against any short-term benefit. Some of the long-term effects of anabolic steroids include increased risk for heart disease, hair loss, acne, liver damage, various cancers, and more.

I never tried anabolic steroids to treat my hives, simply because the side effects didn't seem worth the minor benefit of reduced symptoms. When reading the studies, it seemed to me that Danazol was administered in high doses to achieve a reduction in symptoms. Even so, it was still ineffective for some, and others had a relapse of symptoms.

While this drug has been used experimentally, this isn't a mainstream treatment for this condition. I'd urge anyone with cholinergic urticaria to try other treatments with fewer side effects first.

Corticosteroids

Corticosteroids are not the same as anabolic (muscle-building) steroids. Corticosteroids are a class of steroid hormones that are produced in the adrenal cortex, and it's involved in a wide range of physiologic systems, including the immune system and regulation of inflammation.

Corticosteroids can come in various forms such as creams, pills, or shots. Doctors prescribe corticosteroids to reduce inflammatory conditions such as hives or autoimmune diseases. Doctors also prescribe it in lotion form to help with skin inflammation conditions (such as eczema).

Doctors have used corticosteroids to treat severe cholinergic urticaria symptoms. Prednisone is an example of a corticosteroid that is sometimes prescribed for various immune-related diseases.

It has also been prescribed for some sufferers of cholinergic urticaria due to its immune suppressing effects.

While corticosteroids can reduce the symptoms of cholinergic urticaria, they make a poor treatment option and are not meant for long-term relief. They achieve a reduction in symptoms by reducing the immune system, which can lead to an increased chance of infection, cancers, increased blood sugar, and other health issues—especially if used long-term.

For the most part, corticosteroids should be avoided. They may help in severe cases to reduce the effects of the immune system, but doing so comes with many risks. The effects of this treatment are only temporary, and when the symptoms do return, they may be even more aggressive due to a "rebound effect" that is sometimes experienced when taking corticosteroids.

I've had a corticosteroid shot exactly two times. The first time was when I first developed cholinergic urticaria. I'd struggled for a couple of months, and finally convinced my mother to take me to a dermatologist. He didn't have a clue what was wrong with me, but he could see that my symptoms were real (I had an attack right in front of him!). He first prescribed Hydroxyzine, which didn't work. During my second visit with him, he left the room and came back with a "steroid shot," which the nurse administered into my right buttock.

I was a little concerned about getting the shot. However, after I got home, I thought to myself, "Hey, I'm not going to let this steroid shot go to waste…I'm going to exercise and build some muscle!" Therefore, I exercised diligently for the next couple of weeks. Only later did I realize it was a corticosteroid, not an anabolic steroid!

This shot didn't seem to help at first, although I did experience a remission of my hives a few months later. Whether this was due to the steroid shot, I'll never know. Nevertheless, my hives did come back with a vengeance after a few years, and with them came more aggressive symptoms: skin rashes, stomach cramps, etc.

My second experience with a corticosteroid shot was when my hives were at their worst a few years later. After considering the first shot and hoping that was what set my hives into remission the first time, I tried another visit to the dermatologist. I had to convince them to give me the shot, and they finally did so in my right deltoid (shoulder muscle). However, this did nothing to help my hives.

Overall, I would recommend people not take corticosteroids, especially as a long-term treatment. In severe cases of allergic disorders, they can provide temporary relief. However, they can be dangerous and have many side effects.

Beta-blockers

Beta-blockers block the action of endogenous catecholamines (epinephrine and norepinephrine) on β-adrenergic receptors, a part of the sympathetic nervous system that mediates the "fight or flight" response. They also reduce the heart's rate and make the body feel less anxious and more relaxed (which can help with the emotional trigger of this form of hives).

Propranolol has been prescribed in an attempt to help treat the condition of cholinergic urticaria (hives). Some research articles have reported some success with this treatment, while others found it ineffective. In cases where doctors prescribed this drug, they also prescribed other medications with it

(Source: http://www.redorbit.com/news/health/1273096/successful_treatme nt_of_disabling_cholinergic_urticaria/).

I never tried a beta-blocker because the research articles I read didn't seem very convincing regarding its efficacy in treating cholinergic urticaria. In addition, beta-blockers do have side effects, including dry mouth, sleep problems, diarrhea, and more.

This is not a mainstream treatment for cholinergic urticaria, and I wouldn't recommend it myself based on the lack of long-term success. In my opinion, people are probably less reactive due to the relaxing effect only. Again, if your doctor prescribes this, you may want to talk about any harmful side effects and weigh those against any potential benefit.

UVB Light/Sunlight Therapy (also called Phototherapy)

UVB light therapy has also been used to treat cholinergic urticaria. Some individuals have reported that regular UVB light therapy reduced or even eliminated cholinergic urticaria symptoms while the treatment was ongoing. However, some patients reported that the symptoms returned once the treatment ceased.

(Sources: http://www.cholinergicurticaria.net/uvb-therapy-or-tanning-beds-for-cholinergic-urticaria-treatment/ and http://www.ncbi.nlm.nih.gov/pubmed/2416176)

Dermatologists or skin specialists often administer this treatment using specialized equipment and bulbs, which are different from tanning beds or the sun's rays. With this treatment, there are side effects to consider. Consistent exposure to UVB light can be very harmful to the skin. Risks include increased cancer risks, premature skin aging, skin damage, and other risks. Talk to a doctor to learn more about the risks and benefits of this therapy.

I wrote many times on the website about the possibility of sun therapy to cure or treat cholinergic urticaria. In my own experience, the sun did help me to sweat on some days, but I never experienced longstanding relief from this treatment alone. I never tried a phototherapy treatment in a dermatologist's office, either. I only tried vitamin D supplements and natural sunlight exposure.

My personal views on this treatment is that the side effects and cost of such a treatment would likely outweigh the benefits, especially if a safer or less expensive treatment works just as well. However, in severe cases, this may be an option to consider.

Benzoyl Scopolamine and Oral Scopolamine Butylbromide

Scopolamine Butylbromide is an anticholinergic/antispasmodic medication. Although it's not a common treatment, this has been used to treat cholinergic urticaria because it can help prevent cholinergic activity. In one study, doctors combined it with antihistamines to reduce symptoms in a patient.

(Source: Ujiie, H., Shimizu, T., Natsuga, K., Arita, K., Tomizawa, K. and Shimizu, H. (2006), Severe cholinergic urticaria successfully treated with scopolamine butylbromide in addition to antihistamines. Clinical and Experimental Dermatology, 31: 588–589. doi: 10.1111/j.1365-2230.2006.02117.x)

Like all other treatments, this varies in its effectiveness, and not all people will experience relief. In the study cited above, antihistamines had to be used in conjunction with this medication to reduce symptoms.

This drug does have many potential side effects, so you should always consult a doctor before trying it. Some of the possible side effects include confusion, drowsiness, disorientation, hallucinations, depression, incoherence, dizziness, excitement, delirium, flushing, weakness, memory disturbances, palpitations, tachycardia, postural hypotension, paradoxical bradycardia, blurred vision, photophobia, dilated pupils, difficulty swallowing, and more.

Since the possible side effects alone are worrisome, I never even considered this treatment. When you combine that with the fact that antihistamines had to be used along with it—it just didn't seem like a feasible treatment, especially as a long-term treatment.

For a brief discussion on this treatment, see this link: http://www.cholinergicurticaria.net/scopolamine-butylbromide-for-cholinergic-urticaria/

Anti-Immunoglobulin E Therapy with Omalizumab

This is a relatively newer treatment used in many different types of allergic and asthmatic conditions. This medication works by binding to Immunoglobulin E in the body. Immunoglobulin E is responsible for allergic inflammation. Therefore, this medicine seeks to reduce the number of IgE compounds in the body, thereby reducing inflammation.

There has been at least one study suggesting this could have successfully treated a person with cholinergic urticaria (1). However, there are several reports of this being an ineffective treatment (2).

(Source 1: http://onlinelibrary.wiley.com/doi/10.1111/j.1398-9995.2007.01591.x/full)
(Source 2: http://www.cholinergicurticaria.net/treatment-of-cholinergic-urticaria-with-immunoglobulin-e-therapy-omalizumab/)

Another concern with this medication is the potential for serious side effects, which may include anaphylaxis, wheezing, shortness of breath, hives, dizziness, flushing, abdominal pains, and more. Since IgE may play an important role in the body's detection of cancer, some people have speculated that this could increase your risk for cancer, although this has not been proven conclusively at the time of this writing.

Given the fact that many people have reported this not helping, the potential side effects, and the potential cost, I was never particularly interested in trying this treatment. Many other people with cholinergic urticaria also voiced concerns over the cost and potential side effects associated with it. Therefore, I wouldn't personally recommend it, especially as a long-term treatment. However, it is an option that is available.

73

Nerve or Neuropathic Medicine Therapy

One individual reported some relief (but not a complete cure) with a medicine that affects the nervous system: Gabapentin/Neurontin. This medication is sometimes used in the treatment of anxiety, epilepsy, diabetic neuropathy, and other conditions. It is not a mainstream treatment for cholinergic urticaria, so sufferers may have difficulty convincing their doctors to let them try it.

There is not yet enough data to know if this treatment is effective or safe to use in treating cholinergic urticaria, especially long-term. Gabapentin/Neurontin does have potential for side effects, including diarrhea, vomiting, dizziness, headache, uncontrollable shaking, and more. Given the fact that it does not totally absolve symptoms, it may not be an ideal treatment option.

I never tried this drug personally, and given the side effects, I probably wouldn't recommend it for the long-term treatment of this disorder. If you'd like to see a discussion from individuals who had this condition, see this link for more information: http://www.cholinergicurticaria.net/gabapentin-neurontin-for-cholinergic-urticaria/

Antidepressants and Anxiety Medications

Some antihistamines also have anti-anxiety or antidepressant qualities. Doxepin and Hydroxyzine are two examples of such antihistamines. Doctors often prescribe these antihistamines for cholinergic urticaria due to their combination of antihistamine, anti-anxiety, and antidepressant characteristics. Even so, many are still ineffective in treating severe cases of the disorder.

At least one person has reported an improvement in their hives when taking an antidepressant as a stand-alone medicine; however, others have tried antidepressants without relief. You can read more about these experiences on the cholinergicurticaria.net website: http://www.cholinergicurticaria.net/anti-depressants-doxepin-for-cholinergic-urticaria-hives/

Individuals with cholinergic urticaria may experience bouts of depression, social anxiety, and more. Doctors may prescribe an antidepressant medication to treat any associated depression, anxiety, and related symptoms; however, antidepressants (as a stand-alone treatment) are not a common treatment for this disorder.

Because antidepressants are very serious drugs that can alter thinking patterns and brain activity, I'd recommended that you seek safer treatments first. I have known many people that exhibited side effects from antidepressants, and in some people, they can increase the risk of suicide. My wife and I lost a loved one to suicide, and the individual was on antidepressants at the time. Many studies have shown a link between an increase in suicidal thoughts and the use of certain types of antidepressants.

Potential side effects from taking antidepressants can include an increased risk of suicidal thoughts, weight gain, dry mouth, and more. Again, talk to a doctor about all of the risks associated with this medication, and consider using safer treatment options first.

Hormone/Thyroid Therapy

Hormonal changes can sometimes cause odd symptoms in the body. Some people have speculated that cholinergic urticaria symptoms could be due to a hormone imbalance. There have also been one or two instances of people reporting relief from their symptoms after taking hormone/thyroid therapy; however, this does not seem to be the cause of symptoms for the majority of sufferers.

In cases where hormone therapy did help, the individual had an imbalance in the thyroid levels and/or other hormone levels. After taking the appropriate therapy, they did report experiencing relief. I should also note that other individuals have also reported having hormone imbalances, yet after therapy, they did not experience relief from their hives symptoms. Others have been tested, and their hormone levels appeared normal.

Taking synthetic hormones does have its risks, and this is something you'll want to discuss with your doctor. I'd only recommend trying a hormone therapy if you have a severe deficiency, or if your doctor suggests you do so.

To view the discussion about hormone/thyroid therapy, you may want to read the following discussion of a few sufferers: http://www.cholinergicurticaria.net/thyroid-hypothyroid-or-hormone-imbalance-cause-cholinergic-urticaria-hives/

Leukotriene Receptor Antagonists

Monteleukast (Singulair) is a leukotriene receptor antagonist that is sometimes used to treat asthma or chronic hives. When treating cholinergic urticaria, this medication is often combined with antihistamines or other treatments for the maximum effect.

At least two individuals have reported relief when using Monteleukast in combination with antihistamines or other treatments. It is not a widespread treatment option, but it may be worth considering. You can view the discussion of this drug here: http://www.cholinergicurticaria.net/singulair-montelukast-for-cholinergic-urticaria-hives/.

I never tried this medication myself, but it is often used when treating asthma. It does have some potentially serious side effects, and they should be considered. An example of some of these side effects may include stomach pain, headaches, drowsiness, and more.

Some studies have also suggested an increased chance of getting Churg-Strauss syndrome, a potentially serious autoimmune condition. However, other studies have suggested that this medicine simply unmasked the condition and was not the direct cause.

Treatments that Probably Won't Help Your Hives

In this section, I want to discuss some of the treatments people have mentioned over the years that probably won't help your hives at all. You may ask the logical question, "If these treatments won't help my hives, why mention them?"

First, I want this book to be as comprehensive as possible. This means including things that you may hear about but never try. Second, some of these treatments are silly, and I don't want you to be scammed out of your money. I've probably lost a small fortune in some of my hair-brained ideas over the year. In my defense, hives can drive a person nearly mad.

Third, I don't want you to develop a false hope in some "natural" treatment, only to be burned and left poorer and just as itchy. Some of the websites promoting these products seem very professionally designed, and they have very convincing sales pages.

Therefore, this chapter will cover treatments that are new, likely to be ineffective for this disorder, uncommon, or just downright silly.

Antibiotic Medications

Hives, in general, can sometimes form due to an infection in the body. I remember when I first went to the dermatologist. He stood there looking at me having a reaction, and he asked me, "Do you have an infection anywhere?" I replied, "No, not to my knowledge."

I did find one report online—a forum post on Yahoo Answers—in which a person did describe cholinergic urticaria symptoms. He said he was prescribed a course of antibiotics. It is unclear whether this treatment helped his hives. Nevertheless, I cannot recall ever hearing of a time when taking a course of antibiotics actually resolved the symptoms of cholinergic urticaria.

In fact, I even took a course of antibiotics myself. I developed a sinus infection at one point, and the doctor prescribed me 875 mg of Amoxicillin, twice per day for ten days. If I had any infection in my body, the amoxicillin would have almost certainly knocked it out.

In most cases, doctors can perform a simple blood test to check for signs of an infection. In most cases, you'd know if you had one (pain, swelling, etc.). In the rare case where you might not know, a simple blood test should rule it out.

What's interesting to note is that some have actually speculated that antibiotics could have caused their cholinergic urticaria to develop. Others have reported on the cholinergic urticaria site that they did indeed try a course of antibiotics without success.

If you'd like to see some of the discussions on this topic, this page may be helpful: http://www.cholinergicurticaria.net/could-antibiotics-cause-cholinergic-urticaria/.

In conclusion, there are no reports of antibiotics helping cholinergic urticaria, nor have there been any reports of antibiotics causing cholinergic urticaria. Your doctor probably won't prescribe them for this condition alone, unless he or she suspects you have an infection.

Candida (Yeast) Infections and Antifungal Medications

If you search online for "Candida infections," you're likely to come across a plethora of articles telling you that yeast has overgrown in your body and that your life is doomed. Unless, of course, you buy their homeopath remedy or book (at the very low price of $49.99, I'm sure).

Many people with cholinergic urticaria have fallen victim to this notion, and I'm one of them. There was a time when I strongly suspected that I had a systemic Candida infection. I even spotted some white stuff on my tongue (we all have some naturally occurring yeast on our tongue). I even had all the "symptoms" that the articles suggested you'd have if you had Candida overgrowth (which, by the way, are common symptoms for just about anything).

So I tried anti-Candida diets, I ate loads of garlic, and I even got real antifungal medication (Diflucan). Nothing changed. Many other cholinergic urticaria sufferers have reported falling victim to the "Candida" scam, and they too experienced little to no relief after trying various homeopathic remedies.

Our bodies naturally have yeast inside them. It is on your tongue, in your digestive system, and so forth. A serious overgrowth is rare, but if it does happen, there are real medicines that can treat it quickly.

I should also note that there is a condition that can somewhat mimic cholinergic urticaria, and it is called tinea versicolor. This fungal infection can cause skin discoloration. It can also block sweat pores and cause an itchy condition similar to cholinergic urticaria. However, doctors can treat it with medicine, and although it has some symptoms that mimic cholinergic urticaria, it is a different disorder.

In short, beware of the "yeast overgrowth" movement. If you suspect you have an actual fungal infection, there are very effective treatments for them.

Parasite Zappers

One of the most bizarre treatments I've heard someone suggest for cholinergic urticaria is the infamous "parasite zapper." The Internet is littered with silly products like these, and I've even read some articles claiming that these parasite zappers can cure cancer!

Of course, most of these articles are trying to sell you one for about $100-200. I never fell for this "treatment," and I wouldn't recommend trying it. If you think getting a shock will cure you, I'd gladly shock you free-of-charge.

One of the funniest claims that these people make is that there is a "conspiracy" amongst the big drug companies and hospitals. They want you to come to them, and they don't want you to find out about these amazing parasite zappers. It's all a conspiracy.

What makes that claim so silly is that my wife is a nurse, and I've been to hospitals. My wife and I just recently had our first child, and the total bill came to nearly $30,000 (for a normal, healthy delivery—no complications).

Trust me, if these parasite zappers worked, your local hospital would have a state-of-the-art zapping machine, and they'd gladly zap you. Then they'd send you a bill for about $4,000.

Acupuncture

I've read several people talk about trying acupuncture for cholinergic urticaria. Some seemed to suggest that it only helped a bit, whereas most reported almost no relief over time. I'm not a big fan of these types of "remedies," mostly because I believe it to be ineffective for most medical conditions.

Given the likely high cost and lack of verifiable data suggesting it helps this condition, it would probably be a good idea to avoid this as a treatment.

Nevertheless, if you want to read about some people's experience, you can read a collection of comments on the following page: http://www.cholinergicurticaria.net/acupuncture-ineffective-against-cholinergic-urticaria/.

Herbal tea

While I'm highly skeptical of tea being able to help hives, some have reported that it seemed to lessen symptoms slightly. However, some reported that it made their symptoms worse, too.

My personal opinion is that tea, by itself, will probably not make cholinergic urticaria any better. Nevertheless, you can read more about it here: http://www.cholinergicurticaria.net/could-tea-cause-or-help-cholinergic-urticaria/.

Alternative, Naturopath, and Homeopathic Practitioners

There are myriads of "alternative" or "homeopathic" practitioners on the web who can allegedly help cure various hives conditions. Some even "specialize" in hives. Unfortunately, most individuals with cholinergic urticaria have reported little or no benefit from trying these approaches.

I've even had homeopathic practitioners try to set up accounts on my website in an attempt to solicit members of the forum to their own websites so that they can sell their specialized "services" or "products" to cure them.

Most of these people are all the same: They all suggest you have some "imbalance" in your body. Alternatively, perhaps they'll suggest you have a parasite, a Candida infection, or "leaky gut." The point is that they always have a solution for why you have cholinergic urticaria, and it usually seems logical on the surface. Some even go to extraordinary lengths to write very convincing articles on their websites. However, most of these people are out to take your money.

My approach was always simple: If they were willing send me a free shipment of their product or service, I'd be happy to try it. If it cured me, I'd gladly promote their product free on my website.

81

If, on the other hand, it didn't work, then I'd alert everyone on the website that they are scammy products. To date, I've never had anyone offer to give me his or her product/service free. It seems strange, considering their products allegedly cure hives so well. You'd think they would have been excited about that offer.

In conclusion, I'd urge people to beware of any naturopath/homeopath practitioner using similar sales pitches above. Maybe they aren't all scammers, but they certainly haven't been very helpful, either.

Apple Cider Vinegar

Another product people have mentioned a few times on the website was apple cider vinegar. The idea was that vinegar has amazing healing properties and that it can help treat hives. After having tried it myself, I'm quite skeptical that vinegar can do much of anything for hives.

I've used vinegar on my skin, and I've also drank it. The only thing it did was make me smell like a giant pickle.

Again, you have to be skeptical when dealing with claims online because many people will register for forums and leave comments on various websites in an attempt to promote a certain product.

Nevertheless, you may want to read some discussions on the website:

http://www.cholinergicurticaria.net/apple-cider-vinegar-for-cholinergic-urticaria-and-hives/
http://www.cholinergicurticaria.net/apple-cider-vinegar-for-eczema-cholinergic-urticaria/

Histame/Histamine Supplements

Histame is a supplement containing Diamine Oxidase, an enzyme that breaks down histamine. I first heard about this supplement when a member of the website forum mentioned that he intended to buy it. The idea was that this supplement might help reduce histamine levels in the body, which may lead to a reduction of hives symptoms.

After trying the supplement, however, the person reported that it didn't seem to help. This was only one experience, but I am somewhat skeptical of the supplement with regards to treating cholinergic urticaria. You can always try a low-histamine diet to see if that aids in reducing symptoms. I tried a low-histamine diet, and it didn't completely help me. I realized that many foods that are low in histamine still caused my symptoms to flare.

You can read more about this supplement here: http://www.cholinergicurticaria.net/histame-supplement-for-cholinergic-urticaria-or-hives/

Hives Sprays, Creams, and Ointments

There are some websites promoting sprays, ointments, or creams that suggest that they can treat "heat hives." I have never, in all of my time managing the forum, ever heard of one of these actually working. I won't mention one particular hives spray by name, but the website even has an article directly targeting various types of hives, with cholinergic urticaria being one of them.

I have tried various "sprays" in an attempt to cure this. I purchased one spray that contained "special" oil for nearly $60. It did nothing except made me stink. I've also tried olive oil on my skin, but it did nothing for my hives.

I have to admit that sometimes I get frustrated when I feel people are selling "snake-oil" to people who are suffering in order to make a fast buck. It just isn't right. I don't care if they offer a 100% money-back guarantee or not. They shouldn't give people false hope.

In addition, I may briefly mention that I do run advertisements on my website via the Google AdSense program to help cover the hosting expenses. This program places various ads on my website, and they are usually targeted to match keywords on the page (and sometimes they match items you've been searching).

I try to weed-out any of these scammy advertisements to the best of my ability, and if you ever see a snake-oil product being advertised, feel free to report it to me so that I can block it. I am not affiliated with these advertisements, and in fact, I do not even know who or what may be appearing on the site.

Citrus Fruit

There was one post describing a dried citrus fruit that allegedly helped a person's hives. I've tried various citrus fruits over the years, and nothing has ever helped me. Others on the forum have also commented about trying citrus fruits without success.

I am quite skeptical that this was the cause of any cure, and I have never seen any additional reports of it working. Therefore, I personally wouldn't recommend this as a viable treatment.

Nevertheless, you may want to read the article here: http://www.cholinergicurticaria.net/can-citrus-fruit-or-oranges-help-treat-or-cause-cholinergic-urticaria/

Herbal Remedies

There have been various people register on the forum and recommend an herbal supplement/drink. I promptly deleted most of these posts because it was obvious they were promoting these products in a spammy way, which violated the terms of the forum.

Some examples of the products mentioned include the following:

-MonaVie health drinks

-St. John's Wort

84

-Candida cleanses

-Antifungal treatments

-Acai berries

-Various vitamin supplements

-Digestive enzymes

-and more

While some of the products above may be okay for some things, I feel that these products are not suited to treat cholinergic urticaria. I'd be very skeptical of any claims to the contrary.

Chapter Conclusion

There are various ways to treat cholinergic urticaria symptoms. I've tried to start with the basics: natural ways to treat symptoms or avoid attacks. I then discussed some of the medicinal treatment options used to treat cholinergic urticaria. Lastly, I've discussed some of the less effective or less common treatment options that people have mentioned or tried.

I'd urge everyone to always talk to a doctor, use the least amount of medication as possible (ideally none), and always maintain a healthy level of skepticism towards any products or "cures" you read about online.

Chapter 6: Other Diseases in Relation to Cholinergic Urticaria

Diseases often have symptoms that can match the symptoms of other diseases. This can sometimes lead to a false diagnosis. For example, the common cold has some of the same symptoms as the flu (runny nose, fatigue, etc.), but they are different.

In this same way, other diseases have symptoms that match some of the symptoms of cholinergic urticaria (itching, flushing, and a prickly feeling). Therefore, I wanted to mention some of the diseases that may be confused with cholinergic urticaria.

In addition, cholinergic urticaria is sometimes associated with allergic disorders, including asthma, eczema, seasonal allergies, or food allergies. It is also possible for individuals to have another physical urticaria along with cholinergic urticaria. There have been several posts of people having both cholinergic and cold urticaria.

In this chapter, I'll discuss some of the common diseases that may mimic cholinergic urticaria, and I'll give a brief overview of some of the allergic disorders, miscellaneous conditions, and other urticarias that may accompany it.

Diseases that Mimic Cholinergic Urticaria

Some diseases have very similar symptoms to cholinergic urticaria. It can be easy to misdiagnose the disease for this reason. That's why it is important for a medical doctor knowledgeable about this disease to diagnose you.

Listed below are some of the most common disorders that may be confused with cholinergic urticaria:

Heat Rash (Miliaria Rubra, Crystalline, and Profunda)

Perhaps the disease that is most often confused with cholinergic urticaria is miliaria rubra. This disorder is often called "heat rash" or "prickly heat," which may be the main reason it is confused with cholinergic urticaria, especially since cholinergic urticaria is called "heat hives" or "prickly hives."

Miliaria is a condition in which the sweat pores become blocked and a rash develops. It is common in tropical areas where sweating is frequent. The disease is usually classified into three major types (rubra, crystalline, and profunda), and the classification is based on the level of sweat gland obstruction and the appearance of the rash. Almost every single type has similar symptoms: a "pins and needles prickly sensation." In most cases, a rash is usually present and sweating becomes difficult.

While the "stings and prickly" sensation is similar to that of cholinergic urticaria, there are some distinguishing factors of this disease:

-This disease is self-limiting. It usually clears up on its own within a few weeks. In stubborn cases, antibiotics may be prescribed to help it resolve more quickly. In contrast, cholinergic urticaria is often chronic (meaning, it lasts more than six months), and it usually doesn't respond to antibiotics (I've been on high doses of antibiotics when mine was severe, and it didn't help).

-The rash is usually present. Whereas cholinergic urticaria only produces a rash during a hives attack, people with miliaria normally have a rash present at all times. The rash is very prickly and itchy.

Tinea Versicolor

Tinea versicolor is another disease with symptoms that may parallel cholinergic urticaria. With this disease, a fungus infects the skin, causing the pigment of the skin to change (it looks very similar to the disease vitiligo).

As the fungus eats away at the skin, sweat glands become obstructed. This often results in a "prickly" or "itchy" sensation prior to sweating.

Several factors distinguish this disease from cholinergic urticaria:

-**A fungus causes it**. Unlike cholinergic urticaria, a fungus causes this disorder.

-**Doctors can easily treat it**. Doctors can use a topical agent or antifungal medication to treat this disorder.

-**The pigmented rash is always present**. A rash is easily distinguishable in this disorder due to the pigment changes in the skin. Cholinergic urticaria has no visible rash aside from the hives, flushing, or wheals that may occur temporarily during the reaction.

Mastocytosis/Urticaria Pigmentosa

Mastocytosis (or urticaria pigmentosa) is a disorder in which the body produces too many mast cells. These increased numbers of mast cells can degranulate when irritated, causing an itchy, prickly sensation.

One form of mastocytosis in particular, urticaria pigmentosa, can often produce symptoms that mimic cholinergic urticaria. People suffering with this disorder may experience a prickly, itchy hives reaction when exposed to a physical stimulus such as heat, exercise, alcohol, or stress.

This disorder also tends to leave permanent red or brown "spots" on the skin, which may give a leopard-like appearance. Alternatively, the spots may be very small in appearance and resemble bug bites.

Several factors distinguish this disorder from cholinergic urticaria:

-The red or brown spots are always visible. In contrast to cholinergic urticaria, sufferers of urticaria pigmentosa usually have red or brown spots that stay on the skin.

-The disorder is often present from birth. Urticaria pigmentosa (and other forms of mastocytosis) can present early in life. Cholinergic urticaria, on the other hand, can present at any time, but most commonly appears in the late teens or early twenties.

-The disorder is treatable, but does not go away. In contrast, cholinergic urticaria often goes away over time.

Exercise-induced Anaphylaxis

Exercised-induced anaphylaxis is a disorder that mirrors cholinergic urticaria in many ways. People who suffer with this disorder experience hives, wheals, flushing, and even anaphylactic shock while engaging in physical activity. Like cholinergic urticaria, this allergic reaction ceases when the stimulus (physical activity, in this case) ceases.

Diet has also been linked to a subset of this type of reaction, termed "food-dependent exercise-induced anaphylaxis." However, not all cases of exercise-induced anaphylaxis have been associated with food allergies.

The main distinguishing characteristic of this disorder is that people suffering with it experience symptoms when exposed to an *active* physical stimulus (exercise or active physical exertion), whereas people suffering with cholinergic urticaria can experience symptoms with ***active or passive*** heating.

In other words, individuals with cholinergic urticaria develop a reaction due to any increase in body temperature, whereas individuals with exercise-induced anaphylaxis tend to develop a reaction only during active physical exertion.

Fabry's Disease

Fabry's disease is characterized by a tingling "pins and needles" pain in the extremities, as well as reduced sweating functionality (anhidrosis). The disease is caused by a deficiency of the alpha galactosidase enzyme, which causes lipids (fats) to accumulate in the body.

While this disease only has a couple of characteristics in common with cholinergic urticaria ("pins and needles" and anhidrosis), it has many differences as well:

-There is a reduced life span for people with this disease by 10-15 years. There is no known reduction in life span for people with cholinergic urticaria.

-It isn't curable, but it is treatable. If you have Fabry's disease, you'll have it for life. Cholinergic urticaria is often not a life-long disease.

-No hives form. The "pins and needles" sensation occurs at the extremities and isn't the same sensation as cholinergic urticaria.

Niacin Flushing

While this isn't a disease, flushing due to excessive niacin is worth noting. Flushing is the process of vasodilation, and it causes blood to rush to the skin's surface. This can cause a burning or itching sensation in the skin.

Flushing often happens during a cholinergic urticaria reaction, but it can also happen due to excessive niacin in your diet. Niacin, also called vitamin B3, can produce this "flushing" sensation in the skin when you consume it in excessive amounts. Some people have experienced this flushing after taking certain medications, niacin supplements, or eating a diet rich in vitamin B3.

This flushing, however, is distinct from cholinergic urticaria, as it only happens in response to an excessive amount of vitamin B3 (niacin). There has been no known link between vitamin B3 and cholinergic urticaria.

Allergic Disorders and Other Skin Conditions

Aside from the diseases listed above that may mimic symptoms of cholinergic urticaria, there are also many allergic or skin disorders that may occur concurrently with cholinergic urticaria. In fact, if a person has any of the skin conditions below, they may be at a higher risk of developing cholinergic urticaria.

Since cholinergic urticaria involves the allergic response of the immune system—especially mast cell degranulation—it is also common for other allergic disorders to be present in sufferers.

The list below, while not exhaustive, includes some of the common allergic, skin, or miscellaneous disorders that may accompany cholinergic urticaria:

-Eczema – Eczema, (also called skin dermatitis, skin rash, or atopic dermatitis) is a result of inflammation in the skin. This disorder may accompany cholinergic urticaria. It often presents as red, itchy skin, which often appears around the elbows, neck, hands, knees, and other similar areas.

-Dry skin – Dry skin may also accompany cholinergic urticaria, especially during colder months or in dry climates. I know that I often struggled with dry skin during the winter months, and other cholinergic urticaria sufferers have commented about dry skin issues as well.

-Asthma – Asthma is another condition that is sometimes associated with cholinergic urticaria. Some sufferers have reported having suffered with asthma throughout their lives. Others have reported difficulty in breathing at times during a reaction.

-Rhinitis/seasonal allergies – Inflammation of the nose and mucous membranes (rhinitis) is also associated with cholinergic urticaria. Rhinitis is often the result of allergies such as dust mites or pet dander. In fact, many people on the cholinergicurticaria.net forum have indicated troubled with sinuses.

Allergic responses to dust mites and other seasonal allergies are also commonly reported by people with heat hives.

-Food allergies – Sensitivities or allergies to foods may also be common in cholinergic urticaria patients. While I spent most of my life without major food allergies, I soon found that I had developed many around the same time my cholinergic urticaria presented at age eighteen.

-Acne – Some individuals suffering with cholinergic urticaria have also reported having issues with acne. I've never had this problem, and it may not be a result of the cholinergic urticaria, but it possible that some individuals may be more susceptible to it.

-Keratosis pilaris – Keratosis pilaris is a relatively common skin condition in which small bumps develop on areas of the skin. It is often referred to as "chicken skin," due it is bumpy appearance. It often appears on the backs of arms, legs, and so forth, and it is caused by an excessive build-up of keratin, a protein naturally found in the skin.

Many people with cholinergic urticaria have reported that they also have keratosis pilaris on parts of their body. I have a minor case on the back of my arms, but it isn't significant. The condition itself is harmless, having mostly cosmetic concerns.

-Angiolipomas (or regular lipomas) – While this may have nothing to do with cholinergic urticaria, I thought I'd mention it for sake of reference. I've also noticed several lipomas and angiolipomas on my body. These are small, benign fatty tumors.

They are normally harmless, although I did have one removed and biopsied for safety. I once asked on the cholinergic urticaria website if others also suffered with it, but there didn't seem to be a connection with this and cholinergic urticaria.

Other Physical Urticaria Types

Cholinergic urticaria is only one of the many physical urticaria types. I found it fascinating that so many different urticarias exist, and some sufferers can have more than one physical urticaria type simultaneously. As I mentioned before, a few people have dropped by the cholinergicurticaria.net forum to share that they have both cold and cholinergic urticaria.

Many of these physical urticarias exhibit the same symptoms. The main distinguishing characteristic is that each urticaria type will have a different initiating stimulus. For example, solar urticaria results after sun exposure.

Listed below is a brief overview of some of the most common physical urticaria types:

Solar Urticaria

Solar urticaria, also called sun allergy rash, is one of the types of physical urticaria in which exposure to the sun or other ultraviolet radiation causes a hypersensitive reaction in the skin. This reaction may occur immediately upon exposure to the sun or solar radiation, or it may occur hours later (delayed-onset solar urticaria). Unlike cholinergic urticaria, this disorder primarily responds to solar or ultraviolet radiation—not heat alone.

Solar urticaria most commonly affects areas of the skin that are unprotected by clothing, although some individuals may experience the rash-like reaction even on parts of the body protected by clothing.

When a person with solar urticaria is exposed to the sun, symptoms usually develop rapidly. Symptoms include itching (pruritus), stinging or tingling of the skin, a burning sensation, and small pinpoint hives after direct exposure. In more serious cases (or after prolonged sun exposure), the hives may develop into a large rash of erythema and edema.

Treatments for solar urticaria are similar to that of cholinergic urticaria: Antihistamines, sun protection or avoidance, immunosuppressants, and phototherapy.

Cold Urticaria

Cold Urticaria, also called cold-induced urticaria, is a type of physical hives characterized by a hypersensitive response in the skin after exposure to a cold stimulus. Cold urticaria may appear after direct stimulation with a cold object (such as ice or cold foods), or may occur after a person goes from a hot air mass into a cooler air mass.

When the skin is stimulated with a cold stimulus, hives may develop, along with itching or burning sensations, flushing, small wheals, or localized swelling.

Individuals with cold urticaria may experience a reaction to the following:

-**Drinking or eating cold beverages** or foods can lower the body temperature (or the area around the mouth), causing a reaction.
-**Swimming or bathing in cold water** can cause a reaction.
-**Transitioning from a hot room to a cooler room** (or standing near an air conditioning unit) can cause a reaction.
-**Sweating** (especially if sweating causes rapid cooling of the skin, such as a cool breeze outdoors) can cause a reaction.
-**Getting "goose bumps"** may also initiate a reaction.
-**Handling cold objects** (ice packs, cold beverages, etc.) can cause a reaction.

The treatment for cold urticaria is similar to that of the other physical urticarias. It usually involves taking antihistamines to help with discomfort of itching or hives formation, wearing clothing to prevent the body from becoming cold, etc.

Dermatographic Urticaria

Dermatographism (also called dermatographic urticaria or dermographism) is a skin disorder that is characterized by a hypersensitive reaction in the skin when scratched, scraped, rubbed, or otherwise traumatized.

When a dermatographic urticaria patient's skin is rubbed or scraped, it will often produce a noticeable "red wheal" reaction within minutes. The wheal response that results from direct skin stimulation has earned this condition the name "skin writing disease."

For many people with dermatographism, simply rubbing a coin or stroking a pencil (or other sharp object) along the skin will result in a "wheal" reaction. The person's skin is otherwise healthy and normal in appearance, and shows no symptoms unless it has been stimulated with a sharp or rigid object.

Typically, dermatographic urticaria reactions last between 15-30 minutes before the swelling and wheals disappear. A person with this type of physical hives can literally cause a reaction at any time by simply rubbing the skin with a sharp object (such as a pen, fingernail, knife, etc.). Rarely, the dermatographia may last for several hours.

Dermatographic urticaria treatments are often similar to that of other types of physical urticaria. Antihistamines are often used to control the itching and whealing, and in more severe cases, two different types of antihistamines (H1 and H2) may be used to control symptoms.

People with this condition may also find it helpful to use hypoallergenic laundry detergent, soap, shampoo, and skin care products. Avoiding abrasive fabrics, such as wool, may also be helpful. Keeping fingernails trimmed to avoid excessive skin stimulation when scratching is recommended.

In an episode of the show "Medical Mysteries," they featured a woman with dermatographic urticaria. This woman could take a pin or sharp object, draw a pattern (or write something on her skin), and it would appear in a very distinct pattern.

She said the reaction didn't hurt, itch, or burn. "It just happens," she said. She was always interested in art and wondered what it would be like if she drew a pattern on her skin. She soon discovered that she could draw a pattern, and then the wheals would appear soon after. The reaction would last about 30 minutes.

Fascinated by the reaction, she started drawing intricate artistic patterns on her body. She would then wait for the skin reaction to occur, and when the wheals appeared, she would grab her camera and snap a picture of it.

She then started to display these pictures at art shows. She has since been featured in many art magazines and articles. She has also been able to sell this artwork for as high as almost $4,500!

I guess that is one great example of the saying, "If life hands you a lemon, make lemonade." She turned a bad condition into a lucrative profit and blessing.

Aquagenic Urticaria

Aquagenic urticaria (also called aquatic pruritus, allergic to water, aquatitis hives, or aquagenous urticaria) is a subset of physical urticaria. This type of hives develops after contact with water on the skin. This may include activities such as bathing, sweating, swimming, rainy weather, and other similar activities in which water comes into direct contact with the outer skin (epidermis).

Although it is often described as a "water allergy," it is usually not classified as a true allergy by doctors or researchers. Instead, doctors tend to classify it as one of the physical urticaria types. It tends to be less common than other forms of physical urticaria, such as dermatographic urticaria. It may develop at any age, but most physical urticaria subsets develop most commonly during the late teens or early twenties.

A common misconception is that since the body is made up of significant amounts of water, and since water is a necessity for human life, it is impossible to be truly allergic to water. Therefore, some people may be skeptical of the claims of those suffering with water urticaria. Some even ask the question: "Can you be allergic to water?"

In reality, individuals with aquagenic urticaria do indeed experience a hypersensitive response in the skin after direct stimulation or contact with water. This can be very painful, itchy, or embarrassing for the individual, and he or she can live with the condition for years without being diagnosed for fear of rejection or embarrassment.

Although people suffering from water urticaria can usually drink water safely, they may experience reactions around the mouth if the water contacts the external skin while drinking.

Aquagenic urticaria symptoms are similar to other forms of physical urticaria. Symptoms can include intense itching (pruritus), burning sensation, small hives or wheals, and flushing of the skin in the areas that come into contact with water. These symptoms usually appear within minutes after exposure to water, although rarely the reaction could be delayed by a few hours.

Once the skin is no longer in contact with water, the hives will gradually subside. In many cases, the hives and wheals will disappear within a few minutes. Occasionally, the hives may persist for a few hours after the initial reaction (which is known as "delayed onset urticaria"), although this is not as common.

Treatment for this type of urticaria is similar to that of the other physical urticaria types and may include antihistamines, mast cell stabilizers, water avoidance, UV therapy, and using hypoallergenic products.

Contact, Pressure, and Vibratory Urticaria

Other types of physical urticaria include contact, pressure, and vibratory urticaria. As you might imagine, these types of urticaria are named after the physical stimuli that causes the reaction.

-For contact urticaria sufferers, hives or wheals form when the skin comes into contact with an allergic agent. For many people, this could be something as simple as a new lotion, perfume, deodorant, or soap. Latex, metals, and other similar substances can also initiate a contact urticaria reaction.

-Vibratory urticaria is a hives reaction in response to a vibrating motion on the skin's surface. This can include activities such as playing instruments or using devices that produce a vibrating motion (electronics, etc.).

-Pressure urticaria involves a hives reaction in response to pressure applied directly to the skin. This type of hives may form after wearing tight clothing, a wristwatch, jewelry, and other similar objects that may press firmly onto the skin's surface. A reaction may also occur if a person sits, stands, or lies on a hard surface for an extended period.

These "touch" urticarias are treated in the same way as other physical urticarias: antihistamines and avoidance of known stimuli.

Chapter 7: Cholinergic Urticaria and Exercise

Exercise is important for your overall health. I don't know many people who would dare try to dispute that fact. Exercise helps you maintain good health by reducing your weight, pumping fresh blood to your extremities, reducing the risks for heart disease, reducing the risks for cancers, and so much more. Exercise also helps to reduce the risk for type-2 diabetes and other similar autoimmune conditions.

One of the reasons that exercise is important is that it helps you eliminate fat. Fat is dangerous to your body. One of the interesting facts I learned when I was researching ways to exercise and keep in shape was that visceral fat (that is, the "beer belly" fat) is metabolically active. This type of fat is very dangerous because it secretes hormones that can lead to an increased risk of diabetes and heart disease.

My wife is a registered nurse who has worked in various areas of cardiology, and she'll be the first to tell you that overweight people have far more heart issues as compared to thin people. Science confirms her notions. Study after study has revealed that people who exercise regularly are likely to have longer life spans, an increased quality of life, lower risks of heart disease, and fewer diseases in general. In other words, regular exercise is super important.

However, this brings up an interesting question: If people with cholinergic urticaria develop agonizingly painful hives when they physically exert themselves, how can they ever exercise regularly? Should people with cholinergic urticaria ever attempt exercise, and if so, how should they do it?

How Exercise Helps People with Cholinergic Urticaria

Exercise can benefit people with cholinergic urticaria in several ways. First, you get the ***general*** benefit of exercise that I mentioned above: decreased risk for heart disease, lower risk of other diseases, higher self-esteem, and so forth.

Second, exercise helps you eliminate fat, and if you're overweight, reducing your fat may just reduce your hives symptoms quite a bit. As I said before, fat (especially visceral fat) can secrete hormones that can increase inflammation and worsen autoimmune conditions. If you're interested, you can read more about this in a great article by the National Council on Strength and Fitness (http://www.ncsf.org/enew/articles/articles-obesityandinflammation.aspx).

Another interesting documentary to note is one titled, "Fat, Sick, and Nearly Dead." This documentary takes you on a journey of a guy who was able to improve his health by losing weight. He accomplished this by going on a juice fast. One of the interesting parts of the documentary was a man who suffered with urticarial vasculitis. He tried the juice fast as well, and his symptoms essentially resolved when he lost weight.

If you're overweight, it's time to get serious about losing weight. Even if you can't exercise, diet alone can help you achieve this goal. After all, if you've learned nothing else from having cholinergic urticaria, you should have at least learned that your health is fragile and fleeting. You should do everything you can to maintain and protect your health, and this means maintaining a healthy weight.

Before I achieved my "cure" of hives, I had gained a little weight. It wasn't much (I weighed 170 pounds and was 6ft. tall), but all of the fat was essentially collecting in my visceral (stomach) region, which happens to be the worst kind of fat! This was when my hives were their absolute worst, and losing weight did play a small role in reducing my hives symptoms (although diet played a larger role, which I'll discuss in another chapter). I now weigh about 155 pounds.

The third way exercise helps cholinergic urticaria is that by forcing an attack, it can help release histamine. For people with a mild case of cholinergic urticaria, this histamine release can result in a "refractory period" of up to a day or so, in which the symptoms of hives may be reduced significantly.

In other words, some people with cholinergic urticaria have a regimen where they exercise while enduring the obnoxious prickling feeling that only cholinergic urticaria can bring. If they can persist in the exercise, the hives may slowly fade, and they can sometimes experience relief for several hours (and perhaps even sweat). During this relief period, their hives symptoms may be significantly reduced or eliminated, and they may be able to engage in physical activity with minimal hives.

This strategy works best in people with only a minor case of this disorder. There can be some risks and precautions you need to take if you try this. I'll discuss those in a moment.

In my own experience, this was not an ideal method when my hives were severe. In fact, no matter how hard I worked out (even wearing a sauna suit to try to force out the sweat), I could not sweat or force through the hives attack. When my hives were only minor, however, I did use this method and it would help some.

Precautions and Considerations of Exercising with Cholinergic Urticaria

I'd strongly advise people with this disorder not to exercise until they've considered all of the precautions listed below:

-**Talk to a doctor first**. You should never start an exercise regimen until you first consult a doctor. Your doctor will let you know if he or she feels that exercise is appropriate for you. You should let them know exactly how you plan to do it, how often you plan to do it, and so forth.

101

-Request an EpiPen. An EpiPen is a shot designed to stop severe allergic reactions (anaphylaxis). While not all people with cholinergic urticaria will experience this, there have been a few reports of people going into this type of reaction. This can be life threatening because your airway can close and you may not be able to breathe. Therefore, you should have one of these on hand just in case you ever go into anaphylactic shock.

-Do not exercise alone. Make sure you have an exercise partner with you. Not only can they help spot you (important if you're lifting heavy weights), but they can also dial 911 if you go into shock. Always be sure to have a friend, spouse, or family member with you.

-I don't recommend people with severe cholinergic urticaria attempt this. As I said before, this method is best reserved for people with only a minor case of hives. If you find that your body explodes with hives with physical activity, or if you get hives frequently and severely, this method may only cause you extreme pain.

If you've ever experienced an anaphylactic reaction, or if you have anhidrosis, avoid this method. You may never break through the hives, and you may have a severe reaction. I could have many severe reactions per day when my hives were severe, and no amount of exercise would help.

-Have a backup plan. If your hives do not improve during the exercise, or if you can never break a sweat, consider having a backup plan to abort the hives attack. This could mean jumping in a cold shower, squirting cold water on your body, or anything else. This will help if you experience a severe reaction instead of being able to push through it.

How I Exercised with Severe Cholinergic Urticaria

When my hives were at their worst, I simply couldn't get any sweat out. No matter how hard I tried to endure the hives, I could never sweat or push through the attack. I'd usually give up in defeat and feel even more like a failure.

However, when I finally began my new allergy elimination diet, I also began a new exercise routine. My thinking at this point was that I needed to reduce the small amount of visceral fat I'd accumulated, reduce allergens in my diet, and exercise regularly in order to reduce the severity of my hives. I didn't expect a full remission, but I was hoping my symptoms would at least become more manageable.

Within four weeks, I was able to sweat again. This was the beginning of how I got my hives under control, and over the next year or so, I continued to test foods in my diet and exercise regularly until I achieved complete relief from my hives and discovered what foods to avoid.

Exercise was not something I was looking forward to doing. Imagine that you were held captive in a terrorist camp for a full year, and every time the thermostat inside of your cell reached a certain temperature, you were zapped with the most irritating sensation you have ever felt. Wouldn't it be fair to say that you may flinch every single time the thermostat started edging up to the temperature at which you would be tortured? Wouldn't you also say that you would do everything possible to avoid that sensation?

Well, that's how I had felt about cholinergic urticaria. I did not want to risk putting myself through the worst kind of torture known to man. However, I knew that if I wanted my visceral fat to come off as quickly as possible, I would have to start doing some exercise to burn more calories. So what did I do? I used the "go and stop" method of exercising. Let me explain.

I already had an exercise bike because I had bought one a few months earlier around Christmas. My wife wanted to use one at home, so I bought it mostly for her. I soon realized, however, that it would be a great way to cut out visceral fat.

My first attempt at using it was pathetic. I got the room as cold as I could. It was still spring at this time (near the last week of April 2011), so we still had some cool days in the forecast. I would open the window in the room and turn on a large fan to get it cool. Sometimes I would also soak my shirt in cold water and then put it on. The idea was to get it as cold as possible so that I could exercise for a longer period before my core temperature increased enough to initiate a hives attack.

Therefore, I got on the bike with a mission, and I started peddling very slowly using a low-tension setting. Since the room was really cool (around 59 degrees), I was able to make it about seven minutes or so. Around that time, my hives started to come out with the same intensity as they had in the past year.

To combat this intense reaction, I'd simply stop exercising. I'd wait several minutes until my body was completely cool, and then I'd return and exercise again. That's why I call it the "go and stop" method. I'd go exercise, stop as soon as I got a little itchy, and then go again.

I soon realized that I didn't have to get the full 20-30 minutes of cardio in at one time for it to work. I could break it up in spurts throughout the day, and the exercise still burned calories and counted towards my fat-burning goals. That's exactly what I did. I would exercise for as long as my body would allow–but only up to the point when my hives started itch.

At that point, I would stop and take a long break and cool off (sometimes as long as an hour). Sometimes I would stop a little too late, and have to run into the bathroom to dab some water on my skin to abort the attack. Nevertheless, I would always stop exercising as soon as my hives began itching. I knew better than to push it with my hives being as severe as they were at the time. It just wouldn't have made sense, and it definitely wouldn't have been safe (or fun).

On some days, I could ride the bike for 7-10 minutes at a time. On hot days, I could only ride for as little as 2-4 minutes. Let me tell you—there is nothing that has made me feel as pathetic as only riding a bike for two minutes at a time. Now that was discouraging! However, I did it, and I did it in as many spurts as I could to get my full exercise time in for the day.

Sometimes I would be hopping on the bike a couple of times per hour just to get 2-3 extra minutes in towards this goal. It was rough, but I did this about six days per week, taking one full day off.

After a while, I tried to find other methods to help supplement my wimpy cardio efforts. I began doing any additional exercises I could. What I found out was that for some reason I could work the very lower muscles in my legs with very little effect on my hives. I could hammer my calves with exercises, and it would have almost no effect on my body temperature.

I soon began doing standing calf-raises randomly throughout the day. I would simply go up to a wall and place my hand on it to balance myself, and then I'd lift up one leg (to put all my body weight on the other leg), and then use my other leg (the one touching the ground), to raise up to where I stood on my tip-toes; then lower my foot down.

That exercise works the calf muscle well. I would do several sets on each leg throughout the day to burn a few extra calories. I would also do some "toe raises" sitting flat in bed. While watching movies, I would extend the tips of my toes toward my head, and then point them out towards the end of my bed (as quickly as possible). This works the front of your leg muscles, and after only a few of these toe lifts, the small muscles would begin to burn.

105

Therefore, all day long I would try to find little exercises to do in an attempt to supplement my cardio efforts. I was trying to burn calories any way I could. Those toe lifts can be a great thing to do, by the way.

After about a week or so of doing cardio and a few lower leg exercises, I decided to start implementing some strength training exercises. Again, my hives were on edge, so I was very limited in how long I could do this. I also had to do this in spurts, even when standing in front of an air conditioner.

I began doing a few simple exercises the second week, such as curls for my biceps. I also did a few triceps exercises, squats, push-ups, and a few simple exercises. I didn't use heavy weight for exercises like squats—just my own body weight starting out. I would have to do strength training in the exact way I did cardio–with plenty of breaks.

I didn't let my body get to the point of a severe attack, either. I only did a couple of sets starting out, with as many reps as needed to start to feel a burn. Again, my main goal here was to start stimulating my muscles in a very slow and gradual way, while minimizing any hives attacks. As soon as the hives even suggested they were coming out—I backed off and cooled down.

After about two weeks of exercising this way (and removing many foods from my diet), I was beginning to get discouraged. I still had hives, and they didn't seem to be improving. I began feeling like this whole idea of exercising and eliminating foods was going to be yet another failed attempt to treat my hives. Nevertheless, I pressed on, knowing that I needed to drop a little weight anyway.

During week three, I started to feel a little better. I'd cut many troublesome foods out of my diet, and the result was that my body was becoming less sensitive. I suddenly started feeling much more confident and optimistic. It was a great feeling. By this point, I had definitely dropped a few pounds (nearly 8-10 pounds in about three weeks—not too shabby).

About midway through the fourth week (nearly one month of eating very healthy and exercising daily), I finally had my breakthrough. I was exercising on the bike in my room, with the air conditioner blasting on me. As I sat on my bike peddling away, I began feeling itchy after a few minutes. Like always, I stopped immediately.

For the previous 3 1/2 weeks, I didn't dare try to push my hives. They could whip my butt, and I knew it. So I cooled down very quickly (it was the last cold snap we had in our area before warm weather hit). It was getting late that night, and I wanted to get all of my cardio in for the day. Therefore, after I cooled down a few minutes, I started peddling again.

I was able to exercise quite a while again, and then the hives started. This time, however, I began noticing something that I really hadn't paid attention to thus far—my hives were still coming out, but they weren't itching as severely. Intrigued by this, I kept cycling—but I still didn't want to push myself too far.

Then a miracle happened.

After riding on the bike and dieting for almost a month, suddenly, the prickly feeling faded. When I started to peddle the bike again, it didn't really come back. Only a prickle here and there, but nothing compared to the last year of torture. My hives reaction was stopping while I was still exercising!

I got a rush of adrenaline and happiness by the thought that, since my hives were backing off, perhaps I could actually sweat for the first time in a year. I continued exercising, and I began to push myself. I rode that bike for almost an hour and fifteen minutes straight that night.

When I got off the bike, my legs felt like spaghetti noodles! I reached my hand under my shirt and rubbed it across my chest. To my delight, I felt light dampness. I wasn't covered in sweat, but I felt dampness.

I told my wife and she was elated. "Oh my goodness, your hives are going away," she said. "Don't get too excited. They weren't as bad today, and I did sweat a little. However, I may still have this throughout my life," I replied. I didn't know if this was really working, or if it was just some random fluke.

Therefore, for the remainder of the week, I kept exercising. Each time I would exercise, I noticed my hives were nothing like they used to be. I mean, there was no pushing through them before. However, now I would begin getting very light prickles for a few seconds, and then they would stop. I wasn't even getting the visible hives on my body. I would take a brief break when they started, but I was able to resume exercising quickly. They never got severe.

I was getting happier by the minute. It was as if I'd been a prisoner in my own body for the past few years, and suddenly I was free. My body had changed, and something had happened to make my hives less severe. I was ecstatic but cautiously so.

By week five, things kept getting better. I was still experimenting with my diet and making improvements daily. I was exercising for longer periods on the stationary bike and sweating more each day. My soul was reinvigorated by the idea that maybe this whole diet and exercise thing was actually working.

I was also doing more strength training, and since my hives weren't an issue, I began putting a little more emphasis on building muscle (as opposed to only trying to burn calories). All of this effort paid off. By the end of week five, my hives were barely noticeable. I was sweating vigorously, working outside (physical labor in hot weather), and more. In other words, my hives were gone.

Now I do want to stop right here and make something clear: Exercising and eliminating the small amount of visceral fat I had did help my hives subside. However, what I didn't realize at that point was that the main factor in resolving my hives condition was diet. I was still in the early stages of identifying the foods that offend my body (many foods do this, sadly), but removing the bulk of the inflammatory foods was already helping tremendously.

As of today, diet is by far the biggest focus for me. That's how I know I can keep my hives away. I do still exercise quite a bit, but even if I get lazy and take a month off, I don't worry about my hives coming back (so long as I stay on my diet strictly). However, I do try to stay focused on exercise because it plays a small part in my hives, and it helps my overall health.

Therefore, while I hope this chapter is helpful in explaining how I began to approach exercise when my hives were severe, I hope you also realize that the changes I made in my diet were slowly working to bring the inflammation down in my body, which eventually enabled me to sweat and eliminate the cholinergic urticaria symptoms. The exercise helped remove inflammation, too.

I'll talk specifically about my diet journey in another chapter and explain my current diet in detail.

The Best Exercise Methods

The best exercise to burn fat is aerobic exercise (also called cardio exercise). This is usually preferred for higher calorie burning and other benefits. Lifting weights is also beneficial (especially for strong bones and building muscle), but cardio tends to burn more calories. However, assuming your doctor approves, you should incorporate both methods for best results.

Everyone is going to have a different opinion about the best method of performing cardio exercise. I thought I'd briefly share my own personal experiences/preferences. Also, let me say that you should always follow any advice your doctor or personal trainer gives you regarding exercise.

Walking

There is actually some debate whether or not walking should even be classified as cardio exercise. In my opinion, it shouldn't. Walking can be a great way to ease into cardio exercise, but it is far less effective than true cardio exercise. What tends to happen is that people think walking will help them lose weight—and it will—but only up to a point. Once your body adapts, you will find yourself having to walk longer and longer to continue losing weight.

The only problem with this is that you can burn far more calories doing cardio in far less time. Therefore, if you have four hours to walk every day, then it may work for you. Alternatively, if you are just starting an exercise program, then walking may help get your body ready for exercise that is more rigorous. However, walking is one of the least practical ways to lose weight, get in shape, and exercise for the long-term.

Pros of Walking:

-It can let your body adjust to exercise if you were significantly overweight, obese, have other medical conditions, or just haven't worked out in a while.

-It can be easy on your body if you have some illness/heart problem, etc.

-It can be refreshing to see nature while walking outside on nice days.

-It can be free (unless you buy special running shoes or something).

Cons of Walking:

-You will only see results (in most cases) for a short time. If you think you are getting good results walking, you will probably be amazed at what serious cardio can do.

-It can be bad for people with hives because the weather is so unpredictable. One day it may be freezing, whereas next week it may be 95 degrees. If it is a hot day, you may start itching before you even walk five steps.

-You may be eaten by a bear (hey, it happens), robbed, or endure horn honking or profanities (depending on where you live and walk).

-My wife works in a hospital as a nurse, and nurses walk back and forth for 12-hour shifts, 2-4 days per week, rarely sitting down. Guess what? The majority of nurses at my wife's work are always complaining how they need to lose weight (and many of them are indeed very overweight). Your body is made to walk almost constantly, and you won't burn many calories or fatigue your body doing it–even for 12 hours a day.

-Walking only exercises the legs (unless you move your arms around).

Jogging/Running Outdoors

Jogging or running is a good method of getting cardio exercise. Some people love to run. They're addicted to it. However, the downside is that running (especially outdoors) can be impractical on a regular basis, especially for people with cholinergic urticaria. Here are some of the pros and cons of running:

Pros of Running/Jogging Outside:

-Running is a good method to burn calories.

-Running can be enjoyable for those who like this type of cardio.

-Running is typically free (unless you want to invest in shoes, stopwatch, shorts, etc.).

Cons of Running/Jogging Outside:

-It can be bad for people with hives because the weather is so unpredictable. In addition, it can make you unmotivated to exercise if you have to miss exercise days due to weather.

-You may be attacked by a wild animal, robbed, or endure horn honking or profanities (depending on where you live and walk).

-Running is a little more aggressive on the joints, which can be a problem if you are prone to knee injuries, hip problems, etc.

-If you run in rocky/uneven areas outdoors, you may risk injury by spraining an ankle.

-Running mostly exercises the legs.

Swimming

Swimming can be a great way to exercise if you have cholinergic urticaria. The water will likely help keep your core body temperature down a little longer than other methods. You can still break out in hives while swimming, though (and I speak from experience here). Even in cool water, I've developed hives.

I'm all for swimming, but here is the problem: not everyone has a pool. If you have to visit a gym or local pool, those admission fees can begin to add up quickly, especially if you are going to attempt a 4-6 day per week exercise routine. Therefore, swimming tends to be cost and time prohibitive for most people. Here are some quick pros/cons:

Pros of Swimming:

-It can be fun.

-The water keeps your body cooler longer (which may prolong hives attacks).

-Swimming is easy on the joints.

-You can work out your full body (legs, stomach, back, arms).

Cons of Swimming:

-It can be cost prohibitive/impractical on a regular basis for most people. Also may pose time constraints if you have to travel to a local pool each time.

-There is always a drowning risk.

-You must deal with the weather if outdoors, or deal with people (kids especially) if indoors at a public place.

Treadmills

Using a treadmill can erase some of the "cons" about walking and running. Treadmills can be a great way to get in some cardio, but they certainly aren't perfect. If you love running but dislike some of the cons of running outside, then a treadmill may be your solution. Here are some pros/cons of using a treadmill:

Pros of Treadmills:

-Treadmills allow you to run or walk indoors on your time schedule. This eliminates issues like bad weather, being robbed, or being eaten by a bear.

-It can be an effective way to get cardio/burn calories.

-Some treadmills can fold under beds and/or take up minimal floor space.

Cons of Treadmills:

-They tend to be expensive compared to other cardio machines, with the price usually starting in the low hundreds.

-Treadmills can cause high impact on your joints/knees/hips.

-Treadmills can be one of the more dangerous methods of electronic exercise (countless people have been injured using one).

-Most use a motor, which means it will consume small amounts of electricity. Depending on your electric rate, you may end up spending a few extra bucks per month if you use it extensively.

Elliptical Machines

Elliptical machines are one of the more popular exercise machines. They offer low impact, upper and lower body motions, increased safety (compared to treadmills), and they can be used in the comfort of your own home. The only drawbacks is that they are also somewhat expensive, starting at around $149 for a cheap model.

While I have always felt that the motion was somewhat awkward, my wife loves elliptical machines. We didn't buy one initially, but I eventually bought an inexpensive model for my wife.

Pros of an Elliptical Machine:

-Elliptical machines have low impact on the joints, especially when compared to running/treadmills.

-They take up a minimal amount of space.

-They allow you to exercise both the upper and lower body to burn more calories and give a more complete "burn." This is great because when your legs become fatigued, you can continue your exercise by switching the emphasis to the arms.

-Many people (both men and women) tend to prefer these at health clubs and gyms.

-You can exercise in the comfort of your own home and on your time schedule.

Cons of an Elliptical Machine:

-They can be slightly more expensive than other cardio equipment (roughly the same price as a treadmill).

-I personally feel the motion is somewhat awkward and unnatural, although my wife doesn't share my feelings.

-Some use electricity, whereas others don't. Therefore, some models can increase your electric bills.

Exercise "Stationary" Bikes

This is what I have, and this is what I would recommend. While elliptical machines are a close second, exercise bikes take the cake (in my opinion). They take up the least amount of space, require no electricity, offer smooth and natural motion similar to cycling, are among the cheapest exercise machine you can buy, and most models allow for a full body workout.

Here are some pros of an exercise bike:

Pros of an Exercise "Stationary" Bike:

-They're typically inexpensive. I bought mine for around $100 during the Christmas deals; you can't beat that. They are typically about $120-180 for a decent model.

-You can use it on your own schedule.

-They normally don't require any electricity.

-They're easy on the joints.

-They're one of the safest exercise machines (tied with ellipticals).

-Most models work the upper and lower body for a more complete workout and more calories burned.

Cons of an Exercise Bike:

-Some seats can be uncomfortable when riding for a long time, but you can usually avoid this by adding a pillow or buying seats with extra padding.

-Mine squeaks horrendously, despite tightening and oiling every nut and bolt on the thing. My wife's grandparents also have an exercise bike that squeaks. Go figure.

The Best Type of Exercise Bike

They make many types of exercise bikes (recumbent, upright, fan, etc.). When I bought our exercise bike online, I researched this extensively. I ended up going with a "fan cycle" bike. I would highly recommend you get the same style.

On the "fan cycle" bikes, there is a much more natural motion to riding a bike. The harder your pedal, the harder it is to do so. Some other models, however, don't operate on this same principle, and they offer the same resistance regardless of how hard you pedal.

In addition, the fan cycle bikes have the part where you can use your arms for the back and forth motion, which helps train your upper body. This is a huge help because if your legs start burning or becoming exhausted, you can use your arms for a while. You can keep switching back and forth, and this really gets your heart pumping!

Miscellaneous Exercise

You can also use various other cardio exercises as well. These include everything from a jump rope, various fitness machines, following aerobic videos (such as Tae-Bo or Zumba), and more.

All of these methods are fine, and you should choose whichever method you feel most comfortable doing. Again, I prefer an exercise bike, but there are many ways to achieve a good cardiovascular exercise. Select the method you feel most comfortable with, get a doctor's approval, and have fun.

Sample Exercise Routine

When I started exercising with my hives, I did it six days per week. I didn't follow a specific routine, but rather, I simply did cardio and a few simple exercises when I felt like it (calf raises, bicep curls, etc.).

I usually work out about three days per week now that I have my hives under control. My exercise routine usually involves about 20 minutes of cardio, followed by about 30-40 minutes of weight training.

Here is a sample of what my routine looks like now:

Monday:

I use my exercise bike for 20 minutes, followed by lower body weight training:

      -calf raises (4 sets of 14 reps)

      -squats (3 sets of 12 reps)

      -leg extensions (3 sets of 12 reps)

Wednesday:

I use my exercise bike for 20 minutes, followed by upper body weight training:

      -chest (3 sets of 10-12 reps using flat dumbbell flies; 3 sets of 10-12 reps using decline bench press; 3 sets of 10-12 reps using incline bench press; 1 set of dips)

      -biceps (3 sets of 12 reps of concentration curls; 3 sets of 12 reps of hammer curls; 2 sets of regular bicep curls)

      -abdominals (4 sets of crunches)

Friday:

I use my exercise bike for 20 minutes, followed by upper body weight training:

      -back (3 sets of pull-ups using my own body weight; 3 sets of 12 reps of bent-over dumbbell rows; 3 sets of 12 reps of close-grip pull-downs)

      -triceps (3 sets of dips; 3 sets of 12 reps of overhead triceps extensions; 3 sets of 12 reps of close-grip bench press)

-shoulders (3 sets of 12 reps of standing lateral arm raises; 3 sets of 10 reps of should presses; 2 sets of 10 reps of bending over lateral raises)

Performing the Exercises

Each of the exercises above are done to "failure," which means I use enough weight so that I cannot get the weights back up at the end of the set—regardless of how hard I try. If I can do it, I know I need to increase the weight a bit more.

A "set" is a group of repetitions. A repetition is one complete motion of the exercise. For example, in a bench press, lowering the weight to the chest and then raising it again is one "rep." After 10-12 reps, you'll have completed one set.

If you're unsure of how to perform an exercise, I'd highly recommend you check out some videos online, and/or consult a personal trainer. It is very important that you use the proper technique and form so that you can prevent injury. In addition, be sure to stretch before working out.

I don't follow the above routine rigidly; sometimes I throw in some new exercises or split up my routine a bit. You can mix and match different exercises, and there are plenty of sample routines you can use on the web. However, I find that the one above hits the major muscles, and keeps me in shape.

As I've said many times, always be safe in your approach: Talk to a doctor, use a training partner, consider using an EpiPen, and more.

Even though I exercise quite a bit, I'll never look like Arnold Schwarzenegger did in his prime. My diet simply doesn't allow me to build much muscle, and the human body has limits without using drugs to enhance muscle growth. That's okay, I'd rather be healthy than have huge, bulging muscles.

Chapter 8: Cholinergic Urticaria and Diet

The biggest factor that led to my hives "cure" was diet. I now know that diet was responsible for the majority of my hives symptoms, as well as other strange symptoms I'd been experiencing. To this day, my hives can easily return when I eat certain foods. They also go away when I stay on this diet.

I've included many strategies and tips on how to manage or treat cholinergic urticaria in this book, but those all pale in comparison to eating the right diet (at least, for me). In this chapter, I'll discuss every detail of my current diet, as well as how my diet has evolved over time.

Of course, before you change your diet, it would be wise to get the approval of a doctor or nutritional expert. In addition, I just want to say this: There is always the chance that your hives have nothing to do with your diet. It was a major factor in my hives, but it may not be a factor in yours. Nevertheless, I'd certainly encourage anyone with cholinergic urticaria to test their diet to see if it is having an impact on their hives.

My Diet Background

Oddly enough, I had no food allergies growing up. I ate anything and everything I wanted: chocolate, ice cream, milk, pizza, cereal, nuts, etc. I particularly came to love food during high school. I'd often finish off one of those ½-gallon tubs of Rocky Road ice cream within a day or two. And why not? I was skinny, the food tasted great, and I didn't think anything of it. I even maintained six-pack abs.

Somewhere in my late teens, however, something began to change about my body. Looking back, many symptoms began to appear gradually during that time. I didn't know it at the time, but these were all symptoms of food sensitivities or intolerances.

The first symptom that developed was stomach problems. I'd often get strong stomach cramps, and the pain would be so severe that I'd get goose bumps from the cramps. The pain would be relieved when I finally had a bowel movement, which was usually diarrhea. This didn't happen daily, but it probably happened at least 1-3 times per week.

I never really paid attention to the stomach cramps, and I just reasoned that I ate too much food or had minor food poisoning. Nevertheless, these cramps continued for many months on and off. This all took place when I was around 17 years of age.

When I was 18 years old, something else happened with my body: I developed cholinergic urticaria for the first time. I remember freaking out and not knowing why I had this weird itching/stinging sensation all over my upper body. It was horrible.

The dermatologist gave me a corticosteroid shot, and a few months later, my hives disappeared. To this day, I'm not sure if the corticosteroid shot had an effect, or if my hives went into a remission on their own. It could have been a "slow-release" corticosteroid shot (such as Kenalog), but I don't know what they gave me.

My hives disappeared for a few short years, during which time much of my stomach ailments also ceased. My life returned to normal, and I nearly forgot about the few painful months of hives.

After that 1-2 year period, however, my hives reappeared. The symptoms reappeared gradually at first. I noticed that I got a little itchy when doing some tasks, and then one day at work, I had a bad reaction. This soon brought back all of those memories of my previous encounter with cholinergic urticaria.

Within a few months after this, my symptoms returned with a vengeance. My stomach cramps and diarrhea came back even stronger and more frequently than before. My hives also came back, and a new batch of symptoms came with them: I began to get

120

minor rashes on my elbow, hands, the back of my calves, and the back of my neck. In addition, I also experienced frequent canker sores on my inner lip, my eye began twitching often, and I would get occasional muscle cramps.

If the corticosteroid shot did make my hives better, the rebound effect may have ended up making them far worse. I didn't know what to make of these symptoms at the time, and I didn't realize that they were connected.

The rashes/eczema that appeared on my body looked almost like ringworm in some areas. I bought ringworm cream, and tried everything to get it to go away. I even soaked a rag in diluted bleach and rubbed it on my skin daily in an effort to kill the presumed fungus (don't try that!).

After a few months of trying everything to get rid of the rashes, I got desperate. I began to wonder if maybe the rashes were due to food allergies. This is how I began experimenting with diet. I first removed milk from my diet, and to my surprise, the rashes cleared within a few weeks. Before that, nothing cleared them except prescription-strength corticosteroid cream. I also began to notice that my stomach cramps were severe on the days I ate milk.

Letting go of milk was very difficult for me. It meant I would have to give up all dairy stuff—cereal, ice cream, pizza, and all those other foods I craved daily. I also had many "relapses" during this time. I'd become so frustrated and crave milk so badly, sometimes I'd reason that it was worth the rashes and stomach aches.

I tried everything to keep my milk: eating lactose supplements, trying milk alternatives, etc. Probiotics with lactase helped a lot, but it wasn't enough to eliminate all symptoms. I decided I would have to work hard to stay away from milk if I wanted the rashes and stomach cramps to go away.

A new idea started to dawn on me at this time: Perhaps diet also had an effect on my cholinergic urticaria. This idea launched me onto a long journey of tweaking my diet until I was hives free. However, the journey wasn't easy, nor was it quick.

My Diet Journey

I'd already identified milk as a culprit at this point, so the next step in my diet journey was to cut out gluten/wheat. This was also very difficult for me, but I did it. I noticed my hives seemed slightly better, but the symptoms were still there.

Over the next few months, my diet experimentation continued. I began cutting out more and more foods, hoping that something would cure me. During this time, I began noticing that my hives would definitely decrease in intensity when I avoided certain foods, but they never went away completely. This would often befuddle me, and I'd wonder if my diet was really helping my hives or if it was just a fluke.

I'd often get discouraged, then splurge and eat a pizza (or some other comfort food), only to be on the toilet a few hours later in pain. After a few months of going back and forth with this, I finally did an extreme diet: I ate white rice mixed with canned diced tomatoes, chicken, fruits, and vegetables.

I stayed on this diet for a total of three weeks, and at the end of it, I noticed a significant difference with my hives. I'd still get itchy, but it wasn't as intense as before, and I had a higher threshold for heat. This made both excited and frustrated. On one hand, I knew that my diet was somehow involved, but on the other hand, I was sacrificing so much eating very bland and boring foods—and my hives were still there (albeit, slightly better)!

After this frustrating episode, I took a break from diet experimentation. I couldn't pinpoint the exact cause of my hives, and I was tired of trying. I'd experience intense food cravings while on the diet, and I had a sense of joy and comfort when I could eat foods I enjoyed. Therefore, I avoided foods that caused major problems (milk, etc.), but I still ate other foods.

In the summer of 2010, my hives were the worst they'd ever been my entire life. They got so bad that I couldn't break through to sweat—regardless of how hard I tried. The visible signs of my hives were also dramatic. I'd get hundreds, if not thousands, of tiny red dots all over my skin. Each one stung with a vicious intensity.

Out of desperation, I made an appointment with a dermatologist. I got a corticosteroid shot and tried a new antihistamine, but neither helped at all. My hives were so severe that I couldn't do yard work or even simple tasks, and I became even more of a recluse.

I began to pray hard and think daily of what could be wrong with my hives. I'd spend hours on the web researching ways to alleviate my torture. This led me to many other specific diets to try, and I began researching common allergens, food intolerances, and more. This is also around the same time I began to get the idea of losing weight to help reduce inflammation (as I mentioned in the previous chapter).

I also learned that you don't have to be allergic to certain foods for them to cause you problems. For example, you may lack an enzyme to digest a certain food, and it can cause all sorts of problems in your body. You may not have a milk allergy, but if you lack the enzyme to break down the sugar in milk (lactase), it will cause you all sorts of unwanted digestive issues.

With my new diet experimentation, I began to look at common food intolerances/sensitivities. Here is a brief summary of the ones I considered:

-**Salicylate intolerance** – This is a sensitivity to salicylates. Salicylates are naturally occurring chemicals that come from plants. They help plants survive various diseases. Many foods have some level of salicylates, although some foods are low in them.

At first, I thought this might have been a possible solution to my hives and stomach ailments, but that idea soon proved false. I quickly noticed that many foods that have little or no salicylates, such as oats or cashews, still caused major upsets to my body. Therefore, I quickly crossed this off my list and moved on.

By the way, if you want to know more about foods high in salicylates, you can visit this online resource: http://salicylatesensitivity.com/about/food-guide/

-Low-histamine diet – I also tried a low-histamine diet. The idea was that perhaps foods high in histamine were building unnaturally high levels of histamine in my body, and by going on this diet, my symptoms would resolve. However, even though my current diet is relatively low in histamine, this diet attempt also proved to be futile.

Many foods rated with low histamine levels (oats, cream cheese) also caused rashes, stomach pain, and/or an increased sensitivity of hives. Alternatively, many foods that were high in histamine caused no problems (broccoli, strawberries). Therefore, I quickly scratched this diet off the list.

For a list of high/low-histamine foods, visit this source: http://www.histamineintolerance.org.uk/about/the-food-diary/the-food-list

-Wheat/Gluten-free diet – I'd already been gluten-free by this point, but it's worth mentioning again. Wheat did cause an increase in my symptoms, and removing it did help from my diet. However, I noticed that avoiding gluten didn't cause my symptoms to cease. In addition, I've also tried various "gluten-free" foods, only to experience stomach pain later.

Many manufacturers and listing whether foods contain wheat or gluten, so you can refer to packaging to determine this.

-Yeast – I also eliminated any foods containing yeast, since it is a possible food allergen. This did not cause my symptoms to go away, however.

-Low-sodium diet – One of the things I did find somewhat beneficial was the reduction of sodium (salt) from my diet. It was truly eye opening to realize that the average person consumes far more than the daily-recommended salt intake.

According to the Institute of Medicine, your daily salt intake should be no more than 2,300 mg per day, with 1500 mg being the adequate intake level. Most Americans probably consume 2-3 times this amount daily without even realizing it.

Removing excess salt from my diet didn't stop my hives, but it did make me feel a little more energetic, and I'm glad I learned this so that I can prevent long-term risks of illnesses. A diet high in sodium can lead to an increased risk of heart disease, stroke, and other illnesses.

-Low-sugar diet – I also experimented with reducing my sugar intake. I also found that I was consuming far more sugar daily than what was recommended by the American Heart Association: 36 grams for men, 24 for women. That's pretty much one soft drink per day, and you're at (or over) your limit.

Reducing my sugar has also made me feel much better, but I eat close to my daily-recommended intake. I've always loved sugar, and since I eat such a limited diet now, I allow myself to splurge.

Removing sugar didn't help my symptoms of hives too much, but again, it makes me feel healthier overall.

-Lists of common food allergies – Lastly, I also examined many of the common food allergies: Nuts, wheat, milk, fish, shellfish, eggs, peanuts, and soy. I tried to remove each one from my diet over time. Ultimately, I ended up eliminating all of those things from my diet, and I avoid them in my day-to-day diet now.

My Current Diet

As I experimented with the various diets, I also began my exercise routine mentioned in the previous chapter. I continued to cut calories, reduce salt intake to around 1500 mg or so, reduce my sugar levels, and cut out offending foods.

I eventually gave up on trying to pinpoint my hives to a specific diet cause (i.e. salicylates), and instead, I began listening to my body. If a certain food caused a stomach upset (excessive gas, bloating, diarrhea, constipation, or cramps), I'd cut that food out. If a food caused rashes (itchy bumps on my hands, eczema, etc.), I'd cut it out. If some food caused my hives to worsen, I'd cut it out.

My goal was to reduce my overall inflammation level in my body, and I was going to attempt to achieve that by reducing my visceral fat and cutting out offending foods.

My reasoning at the time was this: I may not have a type-1 allergy to food (that is, an immediate allergic response such as swelling lips); however, I obviously have some issues with food intolerances/sensitivities. These offending foods were apparently causing inflammatory responses in my body (hives, stomach pain, itchy bumps on my hands, rashes, etc.), so my goal was to cut them out.

I thought that if I could remove most of the offending foods, as well as the visceral fat I'd gained, perhaps my body would calm down, and my hives would be manageable. It worked.

What does my diet look like today? I'll post it below, but just remember that you should always consult with a doctor/nutritional expert before changing your diet, especially for the long-term. Nevertheless, here's is what I eat on an average day:

-White Rice (Minute Rice brand)

-Maple Syrup (Great Value brand)

-Sweet Potatoes (unbranded)

-Broccoli florets (Bluebird brand, cooked)

-Turkey (usually Honeysuckle or Butterball brands)

-Bananas (Chiquita brand)

-Strawberries (Great Value brand)

-Blueberries (Great Value brand)

-Water (the only beverage I drink, aside from making smoothies with bananas/strawberries/blueberries)

I consider the foods above to be my "baseline" foods. In other words, when eating this diet, I can expect my hives, stomach issues, and rashes to disappear. It takes about three weeks if I've eaten many offending foods previously, but it always works. As long as I stay on this diet, I have no problems with my hives, stomach, or rashes. I'll discuss more details about these foods below:

> **-White rice (Minute Rice)** – I eat white rice for a couple of reasons. First, it was often listed as one of the least allergic foods on allergy elimination diets. In fact, many doctors recommend rice as one of the first foods you introduce to a baby.
>
> Second, brown rice has the extra grain on it, and it seemed to upset my stomach a lot. Brown rice is healthier than white rice, but I noticed that I tolerated white rice very well—so I stuck with it. It still has protein and calories, and it gives me some nutrition. Moreover, nearly all other grains cause allergic issues (wheat, oats, millet, buckwheat, etc.).
>
> What's odd to note, however, is that some brands of white rice upset my stomach. I bought Wal-Mart's "Great Value" brand of uncooked white rice, and it left a grainy taste in my mouth and caused minor stomach cramps. I tried

Minute Rice and I tolerated it very well. I'm not sure why this is true, as the only difference is that Minute Rice is pre-cooked rice that has been dried. It also says that it is "high grade" rice, so maybe that has something to do with it.

-**Maple syrup (Great Value)** – To make the rice have a taste, I usually pour real maple syrup (not the flavored stuff) on it. Why maple syrup? It was recommended on a couple of websites I read as being less allergic than other sugars. It also has a lower absorption rate into the blood, and it has some minerals in it.

I buy the Great Value brand, which is somewhat watery but actually tastes great on top of warm, cooked white rice. If it sounds nasty, I assure you it isn't. It actually tastes so good that my wife makes a plate for herself sometimes.

I'd like to add one note of caution: It does have a lot of sugar (obviously), so watch your sugar intake. If you're diabetic, you may not be able to eat this.

-**Sweet potatoes** – I really like the taste of sweet potatoes, and they are a healthier alternative to white potatoes. White potatoes seem to cause an increase in my hives symptoms, but I can tolerate sweet potatoes well.

I usually prepare them by peeling them and then placing them in a slow cooker with my turkey. I let it all cook overnight, and the next day everything is ready to eat.

-**Broccoli** – I also tolerate broccoli well. I usually cook this on the stove in a pot of boiling water, or I steam it using a steamer. I eat it when I eat my sweet potato and turkey.

-**Turkey** – I'm not too picky when it comes to brands for turkeys, as I've tried many different brands and I seem to tolerate them all well. The only thing I'd caution here is that you should make sure they don't have any added flavorings, hormones, or coatings (i.e. 'smoked turkey breast').

I buy the whole turkey frozen, and then I thaw it out in the refrigerator for a couple of days. I then take out the neck, gravy packets, etc. and throw it in a "Crockpot" slow cooker. I add some water, throw in peeled sweet potatoes, and I let it cook overnight on "high." It's delicious, and it's one of the healthiest meats, too. Just be sure to check with a thermometer to make sure you've cooked it well enough.

Other meats (red meat, chicken, and fish) do tend to cause my symptoms to flare, so I avoid them as much as possible.

-Bananas, strawberries, and blueberries – These are the fruits I eat on a regular basis, and I tolerate them very well. I buy the blueberries and strawberries frozen (Great Value brand), but I buy the bananas fresh. Sometimes I eat them individually, but I most often eat them in the form of a smoothie.

I take a large whole banana (or two small bananas), throw in about three large strawberries, and about ¼ a cup of blueberries. I add about a tablespoon of water, and then mix it up. I eat about 2-3 of these smoothies a day, and they taste delicious.

Frequently Asked Diet Questions

Here are a few questions people either have asked or may ask about my diet:

How Do I Eat My Diet?

I normally wake up and eat some rice with maple syrup for breakfast. I then usually eat some turkey with a sweet potato and broccoli, followed by a smoothie about an hour later (as a snack).

I eat this as many times as I need to throughout the day in order to satisfy my hunger. It really doesn't taste that bad, and I find that I have adapted to the diet well. If I begin craving some other food, that craving will cease if I go and eat my regular diet.

I also take a probiotic (usually Digestive Advantage) every other day, just to help with digestion. I feel that it does also help keep my immune system operating at a safe level. I take a multivitamin daily, especially since the diet above has very little calcium in it.

I cook enough rice to last me about two days so that I don't have to cook all the time (although some people suggest you should never store rice like this—I've never had a problem so far). I also place my cooked turkey and sweet potatoes in glass storage containers in the fridge, and that lasts about two to three days. Therefore, I only cook about 2-3 days per week.

When I have to go places, I pack it in a lunch box and warm it up there. It's a pain sometimes, but totally worth it.

Why Does the Diet Work?

I have no idea why the diet works—I just know that it does work. Perhaps I lack some enzyme to break down a certain chemical, and the diet above is very low in that chemical. Alternatively, perhaps my immune system is just hypersensitive to the proteins found in many different foods.

Ultimately, I don't know why the diet works, and that is somewhat frustrating. It's kind of like having a TV that gets fuzzy reception, yet it suddenly works fine once you go up and whack it on the side. You don't know why the TV suddenly works (perhaps an electrical component was jarred back into place); you just know hitting it works. In that same way, I don't know why the diet works, but it does work great for me.

How Long Did I Have to Stay On It to See Results?

When I had a lot of inflammation in my body, it took about four weeks on the diet for my cholinergic urticaria symptoms to disappear. It happened very gradually. Now that I eat the diet regularly, I can sometimes eat foods that cause only minor problems, and it usually only takes a week or so for my symptoms to subside (if they come back at all). My symptoms stay gone as long as I stay on the diet strictly.

How Can You Live Like This?

As tough as this diet can be, it is a walk in the park compared to living in misery with cholinergic urticaria. I'm quite used to it now, although I still do have cravings from time to time.

I went through a rollercoaster of emotions when I first went on this diet. It takes a lot of discipline, and I've failed many times—especially at the beginning of my diet trials. I've had days when I had strong cravings for certain foods, and I'd sometimes splurge and eat them. Then I felt as if I had to start all over again. It was tough.

I've also had days of depression where I felt that even though my hives were gone, my life was still miserable due to this diet. My wife was always great about giving me a "pep talk" so that I'd stop feeling sorry for myself, however.

Is this Diet Safe Long-term?

I have no idea if this diet is safe long-term, and that's why you should consult a diet expert to determine if it is safe for you. Many of the foods I eat are healthy, but I don't eat a wide variety. It's possible I do miss some nutrition. I try to supplement this with a daily multivitamin, and I do occasionally splurge and eat a slightly wider range of foods.

Do You Ever Cheat on Your Diet?

Yes and no. I've learned that there are some foods that cause too much of an allergic response in my body, and I have to stay away from those—probably for the rest of my life. The main offenders are milk/dairy, wheat, and nuts. I also discovered that corn was causing inflammation (in the form of itchy bumps on my elbow) about six months ago. I also avoid foods with a huge ingredient list, as I've learned these usually cause major issues (they usually have multiple allergens, dyes, and preservatives mixed in).

There are some foods, however, that I can eat as long as I eat them in low amounts and stop. Some foods I sometimes "cheat" with include veggie chips, white potato chips, salads (with Italian dressing), craisins, kiwi fruit, natural fruit rollups, rice noodles with diced tomatoes and Italian dressing, and more. I sometimes eat carrots, squash, zucchini, cucumbers, and other vegetables as well. Rarely, I'll cook a pie or cookies using gluten-free flour.

However, I eat these foods only in very low amounts, and I must have long breaks between them if I don't want my symptoms to come back. For example, I may eat a half a bag of veggie chips on the weekend, and then I probably won't eat another snack until the next week. As long as I eat only one "low offending" snack per week, I can usually splurge without my symptoms returning. If I eat these foods too often, my symptoms can slowly return, usually in the form of slight prickles when exercising. When this happens, I return to my strict diet and the symptoms go away within a week or so.

132

Are You Sure the Diet Helps?

Absolutely—I've now been on this diet for about three years, and I've had plenty of time experimenting. I've gone back to my old diet at times, and my symptoms returned. Each time this happens, I simply return to my "baseline" diet, and my body returns to normal.

There is no doubt in my mind (or my wife's mind) that diet was the biggest factor in my hives.

Can this Diet Help Others with Cholinergic Urticaria?

If this diet helped one person with cholinergic urticaria (me), it makes sense that it could potentially help others. However, everyone is different, and there may be different subtypes of cholinergic urticaria. You may even have different food sensitivities.

Alternatively, food may not have anything to do with your cholinergic urticaria, and it could have a very different cause.

The good thing about diet is that you have to eat anyway, so it will cost you nothing—you simply cut out foods and try eating different ones for a while.

A food diary can help tremendously, and you should be on the lookout for any foods that cause an increase in inflammation (allergic response), such as sneezing, eczema, stomach upset (bloating, diarrhea, constipation, cramping), increase in hives severity, etc.

If you try my "baseline" diet and you don't see results within a month, then either you are still allergic to some of my "baseline" foods, or diet is not a factor in your cholinergic urticaria.

Will I Ever Be Able to Eat More Foods?

It's hard to say if I will have to stay on this diet for my entire life. There's always a chance my body will change, and I'll be able to eat the foods I used to enjoy. However, there is also the possibility that I'll always have to eat like this to keep my symptoms in remission.

Do You Feel Any Symptoms When You Stay On This Diet?

When I eat this diet strictly, my symptoms disappear. I can exercise and break a complete sweat without having any hives or itching. It stays this way so long as I stay on my diet strictly.

If I eat moderately offending foods outside of my "baseline" diet, symptoms may return. However, they usually aren't severe, and they seem to go away quickly when I clean up my diet.

Even when "cheating" with too many foods outside of my "baseline" diet, my hives have never returned to the severity they were a few years ago—primarily because I know what foods cause the most problems, and I avoid them.

Do You Add Any Seasonings When You Eat?

No. When I eat my turkey, broccoli, and other foods, I do not add any sauces, creams, salt, pepper, or anything. I eat it completely plain.

Should Ask My Doctor about an Allergy Test?

Allergy tests can be very beneficial for pinpointing common foods that may initiate an allergic response. If you can afford to have one done, it may help you identify troublesome foods that may intensify your hives symptoms.

However, an allergy test may not be able to determine all foods that can cause problems. In addition, allergy tests typically won't pick up any food intolerances—they only tend to recognize actual food allergies.

Therefore, my personal opinion is that they can be beneficial in helping you identify troublesome foods, but you shouldn't rely solely upon an allergy test.

What is the Difference Between a Food Allergy and Food Intolerance?

The main difference between a food allergy and food intolerance is that a food allergy involves the immune system directly (typically IgE). In this situation, your immune system actually builds antibodies against a particular food protein. Thus, when you eat a food that you are allergic to (such as peanuts, shellfish, etc.), there is an immediate reaction (you usually react within minutes or hours).

These reactions can often be fatal in severely allergic situations. There are also non-IgE mediated allergies, such as allergic eosinophilic esophagitis, gastritis, or gastroenteritis. Celiac disease is also sometimes classified as a food allergy since it involves the immune system, but it is also referred to as an intolerance.

Food intolerances are reactions that occur due to the body not being able to tolerate a certain food or substance. This is usually a very slow reaction (taking hours, days, or weeks to show up or go away), and a food intolerance can develop for a number of reasons, including:

-Lack of enzymes to break down a certain substance (i.e., lactose intolerance)

-The result of food poisoning/bacterial disruption in the digestive system

-Non-allergic sensitivities (pharmacological in nature)

Food intolerances, like classic allergies, can also form at any age during life. For example, I used to be able to consume milk with no problems at all. However, in my 20's, I developed lactose intolerance.

Is Your Diet the Same as an Allergy Elimination Diet?

There are various "allergy elimination diets" used by nutritional experts in an attempt to resolve food allergies in patients. However, I developed this diet after researching and experimenting over a long period.

If you plan to try this diet (or another allergy elimination diet), always do so under the supervision of a qualified medical professional. I also highly recommend you keep a food diary so that you can determine which foods may be causing an allergic response.

Most allergy elimination diets involve going on a strict diet until symptoms resolve, and then reintroducing foods one at a time to identify troublesome foods. At this point, I've identified that most foods are troublesome for me, and I'm quite limited on what I can eat if I want my hives to stay away.

I would like to add one note, however. If this diet does work for you, remember that you don't always have to follow it 100%. You can work over time to try new foods, and you can always "cheat" on occasions if you get too overwhelmed. At least you'd know the major cause of your symptoms, and you'd have some control over them.

On the other hand, if you try this diet and it doesn't work, at least you can rule it out as a major factor in your hives, and explore other treatment options to manage it effectively.

Chapter 9: How I Cured My Cholinergic Urticaria

Now that I've discussed various treatments I've tried, as well as how my exercise and diet eventually led to a resolution of my hives, I want to briefly summarize exactly how I've achieved my "cure" from cholinergic urticaria (by God's grace, of course).

The original idea with this "cure" regimen was that it should help decrease any sources of inflammation that made my hives severe. I try to think of it like this: Imagine that you have a slight allergic response to 10 different foods, as well as allergies to pets and pollen. You'd probably be miserable with a stuffy nose, rashes, and everything.

If you cut a couple of the allergic foods out, you'd feel a little better over time. If you cut half out, you'd feel a lot better. If you cut out the pet allergens, you'd feel even better. If you cut them all out, you'd feel fantastic, mainly because the allergic response in your body would have diminished significantly.

What I've found is that many things can increase inflammation in my body. When this happens, my cholinergic urticaria symptoms begin to appear or worsen. When I remove sources of inflammation (foods, products, etc.), the inflammation decreases to the point where my hives are no longer present.

As I've already stated, my hives go away as long as I maintain this regimen. If I stray from my diet, my hives usually return. In addition, while diet is by far the biggest factor in my hives symptoms, I do feel that other things below do help in reducing overall inflammation.

-Diet – Again, this is the biggest factor in keeping my hives in remission. My baseline diet consists of white rice with maple syrup, turkey, sweet potatoes, broccoli, strawberries, blueberries, and bananas. As long as I stay on this diet, my allergic issues resolve.

I can occasionally eat other foods, but only foods that I know cause minimal allergic responses in my body. I must keep a close watch on my diet at all times if I want to maintain a remission of my hives. You can read the details in the chapter on "Cholinergic Urticaria and Diet."

-Exercise – Exercise can reduce inflammation, boost your self-confidence, and help you maintain sweat functionality. I try to exercise at least three times per week, although I do take breaks. Exercise isn't the biggest factor for my hives staying in remission, but I feel like it is a good habit to stay in for health reasons. It also does help reduce inflammation in the body. Moreover, it feels so good to break a sweat again, so that also motivates me to stick with it.

-Hypoallergenic products – I try to use as many hypoallergenic products as I can, just to rule out any chances of being allergic to any chemicals the products may contain. This includes soap (Dove Sensitive Skin), lotion (Eucerin Calming Crème), laundry detergent (All Free Clear), bedding sheets (pillowcase and bed covers that resist allergens), Arm & Hammer deodorant (aluminum free), and so forth.

I do use some non-hypoallergenic products without issues, such as toothpaste and Aussie shampoo. Nevertheless, I do not use any skincare products beyond those already mentioned.

- Probiotics and vitamins – As I've mentioned previously, I do take a daily multivitamin (Centrum brand). I also take different brands of probiotics, although I usually take them every other day. The brands I've tried include Culturelle, Align, Digestive Advantage, and Enzymatic Pearls.

Probiotics probably won't cure anyone's cholinergic urticaria symptoms, but they do make a noticeable difference in the allergic response in my own body—enough that I feel it's worth it to continue taking them. They allow me to eat an occasional "cheat" snack without dramatic symptoms. They also help with digestive health.

-Healthy lifestyle – It is incredibly important to maintain a healthy lifestyle if you want to enjoy good health.

I remember hearing a story about an old-looking man whose face was covered in wrinkles. He had age spots on his skin, he was missing half of his teeth, his hair was thinning, and he just looked horrible. He had to struggle just to get up out of his chair, and he walked with a cane.

A young man came up to him and said, "I heard that you've lived a wild life—you had a different woman every week, you smoked three packs of cigarettes a day, and you drank like a fish. How have you managed to live so long doing all of these things?"

The old-looking man replied, "I'm just lucky, I guess." Then the young man asked him, "How old are you, anyway?" The old-looking man replied, "25."

That's a funny story, but there's a lot of truth in it. Living a rough lifestyle and doing drugs will age you dramatically (assuming you don't die first). I don't want to sound preachy, but I've had many friends and family members who have had their lives messed up by drugs.

Obviously, your body is made of chemicals, and if you put the wrong chemicals in it, it can devastate your health. You can't expect that you can do recreational drugs and experience no health consequences. The laws of physics will not overlook you.

I always hate to hear of people overdosing on drugs or having their lives ruined by them. I just hate it. I've said this before and I'll say it again: If you learn nothing else from cholinergic urticaria, you should at least learn that your health is fragile. You should do everything you can to preserve your health while you can.

I know that I do the best I can to maintain a healthy lifestyle. I get between 8-10 hours of sleep on an average night. I work hard to maintain a healthy weight. I don't smoke, drink, or do any recreational drugs. I'm faithful to my beautiful wife, and I'm not really into any risky endeavors.

I'm not perfect, and I've certainly fallen short many times in my life. However, this condition has been a wake-up call to me about my long-term health. I'd strongly urge you to stay away from drugs if you plan to live a long life (all other things being equal). Please take care of your body; it's the only one you have. I want you to enjoy great health.

Final Words on My Cure

Those things listed above all work together to help me reduce the allergic response (inflammation) in my body. I've tried to be as detailed as I possibly know how to be, and I've expanded on most of those topics above in other chapters. In addition, I have a list of the products on my website here for fast access: http://www.cholinergicurticaria.net/products/ .

Can the "cure" mentioned above work for you? I have no idea. It may or it may not work for you. I discovered it over a period of almost a decade, and I finally found what worked for me. Perhaps you'll have to eat different foods than me. Alternatively, perhaps diet isn't a big factor with your cholinergic urticaria symptoms. It's hard to say. Nevertheless, I am so thankful that I've been able to overcome this disorder, and I sincerely hope this book helps you.

Since overcoming my hives, I can finally live again. It took many months of getting used to the idea that I don't have to avoid certain activities anymore. I don't have to worry about going outside and working on a hot day. I don't have to avoid exercise. I can actually be social when I want and attend church without fearing an attack.

I pray that what works for me works for you. If it doesn't, I hope that other material in this book can help you come to a place where you can better manage your hives symptoms.

Chapter 10: Getting Motivated and Staying Positive

Living with a disorder where you erupt in painful, stinging hives can be difficult. When I first developed cholinergic urticaria, I had a difficult time coping with the changes it brought to my everyday life.

I'd often go through bouts of depression and negative thinking. I can recall many times crying myself to sleep, hoping I simply wouldn't wake up. I'd often say things like, "Why do I have this condition? What did I ever do that was so bad that I deserved it? I wish I'd just die!"

I had this disorder for so long, and with such little relief, that I was miserable. I loathed my life on most days, and I had a very hard time staying focused on other things in my life. My wife would even get restless some days due to my frustration with the disorder, as well as my constant complaining and negativity about it.

However, there is one thing I learned through all of my negativity, whining, and anxiety: It didn't help a thing. Being negative didn't cure my hives. Being negative didn't motivate me to be better. Being negative didn't make my quality of life any better—it made it worse. Negativity only made each day that much harder to get through.

The late motivational speaker Zig Ziglar used to say, "Positive thinking will let you do everything better than negative thinking will." I've found that to be so true. No matter how bad your hives get—or how bad life seems—you must stay positive.

In this chapter, I'll offer you some ways I've learned to crush negative thinking in my own life, and how I've been able to stay motivated and keep moving forward—hives or no hives. I hope they help you overcome any negative thinking or depression you may experience.

Controlling Negative Thoughts

We all have negative thoughts from time to time, but how we deal with those negative thoughts can make or break our attitude. Charles Swindoll once said, "Life is 10 percent what happens to us and 90 percent how we respond to it." No matter what happens to you—a chronic hives disorder or anything else—you, and you alone, control how you will respond to it.

The choice is yours: You can drown in your own self-pity for the rest of your life (as I did for a great while), or you can decide that you're not going to let anything beat you down. You can pick yourself up, dust off your clothes, and decide that you're going to live a positive, happy life. Regardless of your circumstances or health, you can choose to live a happy life and have a positive attitude.

Here are some tactics to squash any negativity that may enter your mind:

Convert Negative Thoughts into Positive Thoughts

When a negative thought enters your mind, immediately think of a way to convert it into a positive thought. I like the old saying, "When life hands you a lemon, make lemonade." Try to approach life with this attitude.

You can convert any negative thought into a positive thought. I've learned this, and it has helped me to avoid those small depressing ruts I used to get into. When you think to yourself, "This hives condition sucks so badly," immediately add to that thought, "But at least it should go away or improve one day. At least I can learn to manage it over time. I'll beat it."

When you think to yourself, "This will never go away, and I'll be tortured with this forever!" remind yourself that I also said the same thing, and today my hives are gone.

A couple in my church recently moved into a new house. One morning they got up, took a shower, and ate breakfast. As they went downstairs to leave, they realized their entire basement was flooded. Apparently, a pipe had started leaking as they took the shower, and all morning it gushed and flooded their entire basement.

They quickly called a plumber, only to find out that he'd have to remove the entire shower for the repair. The woman's response to the whole thing was amazing. She simply replied, "Well, at least I'm getting a new remodel!"

If you think diligently, you can always find a hidden blessing in any difficulty. When I look back at my own experience with this disorder, blessings abound. My hives led me to a place of emptiness and brokenness, and this led me on a spiritual quest to determine if God really did exist. The result is that I eventually came to faith in Christ, which totally and radically changed my life for the better.

Having severe hives also helped my financially. I had to think outside of the box to find ways to make money, as most traditional jobs weren't feasible while my hives were so severe. This led to me starting my own business, where I was able to build websites, write, and other things.

In many ways, cholinergic urticaria nearly destroyed my life. In other ways, it was a great blessing—although it certainly didn't seem like it at the time.

When you feel that life simply isn't worth living, remind yourself that it *is* worth living. There is always hope for tomorrow, and as long as you're still here, there is a plan and purpose for your life. You were created for a reason, and you've been placed in this world for a reason.

Moreover, you can find a blessing in any difficulty. It may not be obvious; you may not even see it for years. Nevertheless, I

145

guarantee you that you can find a blessing in your suffering if you look hard enough.

Count Your Blessings and Answered Prayers

Another way to squash those negative thoughts is to sit down and count your blessings—literally. On days I'd feel really down, I would sometimes stop and try to name every good thing that has happened in my life. I'd thank God for my wife, home, material possessions, wife's health, and so forth.

I'd even stop and reflect on all the stuff that could have happened to me in my life. It's a miracle that anyone lives long in this world. Considering all of the diseases, crime, potential accidents, and so forth—you're practically a walking miracle if you live past age ten.

When you count your blessings, you soon begin to realize that you've been blessed in many ways. This can help diminish and deter those negative thoughts and put things into a proper perspective. You don't have it that bad. In fact, you probably have it much better than most people do.

Aside from that, I'd try to remind myself of all of the prayers God had answered in my life up to that point. I often tell my wife that she is one of the greatest examples of answered prayer in my life. Despite dating often in high school, I never really connected with any girl. I often felt as if "true love" was a farce, and that it was only something you read about in movies or romance novels.

I can recall going to bed at night during high school, praying that one day I would meet a girl that I could fall in love with. I couldn't imagine what it might be like to love a girl in that way—what it would be like living with your mate, and so forth.

Sure enough, I met my wife a few years later (at a time when I'd pretty much given up on the idea of love), and she is my very best friend in the whole world. We've been married for 8 years now, and we couldn't be happier. We love each other with a deep and sweet love—we're inseparable.

Many times when I've felt as if my hives would never get better—or that my business wouldn't succeed—I've stopped and considered the other times in my life in which I felt like that. Those times now seem like a distant memory since God answered those prayers.

Recalling all of the other times in my life in which God fulfilled my desires or answered prayers has often helped me find the energy to get through another day.

Remember that Everyone Suffers

It's easy to think that you've been robbed in life and that everyone else has it easy—not so! The truth is that we all suffer. There's no one in this world exempt from suffering, and no one is getting out of this world alive.

Some people seem like they have it together, but in reality, they are suffering (or about to suffer) with something. We live in a crazy world, and we all suffer together. We all have our thorns to bear. Just think of all the diseases or medical conditions people suffer with: blindness, multiple sclerosis, diabetes, autism, cancer, heart disease, kidney failure, etc.

Some of the healthiest people you'll meet may be on the verge of getting some new disorder or health scare. Someone may seem to have the perfect life, but perhaps they're about to find out their spouse has been cheating, or a loved one is about to die. Alternatively, maybe they are suffering with anorexia behind closed doors—living in misery even though they look perfectly healthy to everyone else.

Some of the wealthiest people you'll meet are miserable. I recently read of a very wealthy man who committed suicide. It reminded me of a quote by Zig Ziglar: "Money won't make you happy, but everyone wants to find out for themselves."

The man had millions of dollars and great status, yet that wasn't enough to make him happy. If you place your happiness upon an external *thing* (money, health, love, etc.), you're only setting yourself up for failure once that *thing* is no longer here. Instead, place your joy in what you already have that can never be taken away, not in the things you don't yet have or that can be taken away.

Yes, cholinergic urticaria is a horrendous condition, but it's rarely fatal. Yes, it hurts, stings, and itches, but it usually goes away or gets better over time. No, there may not be a "cure" in the traditional sense, but there are many ways to treat it, and you can fight to have a normal and happy life.

Negative thinking may bog you down from time-to-time. Learn to crush those negative thoughts, and listen to the positive ones. Choose to think positively, and learn to be content in any circumstance—rich or poor, healthy or afflicted, loved or grieved.

Finding Motivation When You Have None

Aside from dealing with negative thinking, you may also have difficulty getting and staying motivated. I've often found that I had this problem—even on the days in which I didn't feel frustrated or depressed about my hives.

Here are a few tricks I've learned to boost my motivation when I felt like I had none.

Remember that Life Can Change Instantly

One of the glorious truths about life is that it's always changing; it never stays the same. Another great truth is that life can seem hopeless, bleak, and pointless one day, yet your life could take a turn in a completely different direction the next.

Many people have experienced this amazing turnaround in their lives, and the same could easily happen for you. There are many documented cases of people having been diagnosed with deadly cancer and given only months to live, only to be stunned when they returned to the doctor and the scans revealed that the cancer had vanished. It's not common for that to happen, but it does happen.

Sharyn Mackay is one such person who experienced this phenomenon. After being diagnosed with inoperable and incurable cancer—and given only months to live—she later returned to the doctor to find that her cancer had vanished.

(Source: http://www.dailymail.co.uk/health/article-1172211/The-miracle-survivor-I-given-months-live--terminal-cancer-vanished.html)

These stories of health "miracles" fascinate me. It reminds us all that miracles can and do still happen. However, life can change in many ways, and the change isn't always related to health. Any aspect of your life could change for the better in an instant.

For example, perhaps you're flat broke and in a dead-end career. Many of the world's billionaires were also in the same position at one time. John D. Rockefeller, one of the wealthiest men in the history of the world, did not come from a wealthy family. The only education he received was a short bookkeeping course after high school.

John's mother was a devoutly religious homemaker, whereas his father was a fraud who'd spend his days trying to sell phony "cancer cures" and other "miracle" remedies. They both had a profound influence on him—John took up his mother's faith and hard work values, whereas he learned a few savvy business skills from his father.

When John turned sixteen years old, he set out to find his first job. It took him many weeks of trying to find one, but it didn't stop his hunger. For six days per week, John would wake up, dress in a full suit, and walk all over town filling out job applications.

Eventually he landed his first job as a bookkeeper in a local business. This job didn't last long, however, and John eventually left after he didn't get his desired raise. He then joined up with a friend and started a produce commission business—a business that only had moderate success.

Something else soon caught John's eye, however, and he soon left the produce business for a new venture: oil. John went on to start Standard Oil, one of the largest businesses of his day. His wealth grew to astronomical amounts—and he used this wealth to help many churches, hospitals, charities, and so forth.

The point I'm trying to make is that life has a way of changing— sometimes overnight. Even when your life seems bleak, you might be surprised at what lies just around the corner for you.

Are you living life defeated, or are you living life with vigor? Do you mope around all day in depressive ruts and negative thinking patterns, or are you waking up every day with a positive and motivating spirit, hoping that "today" will be the day your life takes on a new direction?

Listen to Others Who Have Persevered in Life

Another thing that has helped me stay motivated is listening to others who have persevered. I love true stories of triumph: stories of "rags to riches," or stories of people overcoming seemingly insurmountable obstacles to achieve something great.

One of the greatest stories of triumph I've ever witnessed during my lifetime is the story of Nick Vujicic. Nick was born in Australia, but unlike most babies, he was born without any arms or legs.

As you can imagine, Nick has to have personal care around-the-clock by parents and caretakers. Even simple tasks that you and I take for granted every day—feeding ourselves, bathing, using the bathroom—is a great challenge for Nick. Growing up, it was virtually impossible for him to do those things without the aid of a caretaker.

He experienced ridicule in school, and soon found himself facing negative thoughts regularly. He would often think thoughts like, "No girl will ever love a freak like me. I'll never be able to have a career—I can't even scratch my own back. I'll probably never have children, and even if I did, I could never even hold my own child in my arms. My birth was a mistake, and I wish I'd never been born. I guess God made a mistake when He made me."

At one point, Nick even attempted suicide by rolling his body over in a tub of water so that he was face-down. However, at the last minute he decided against it, as he couldn't bear the thought of his mother living with the heartache of his death.

Nick Vujicic obviously has a major "disability." No sane person would point a finger of accusation at him and blame him for going on welfare, waving a white flag, and simply giving up on life. However, living with that attitude was simply unacceptable for Nick. While he realized that he couldn't change his circumstances, he knew he *could* change his attitude.

Nick made a bold decision that he wasn't going to give up on life. To date, Nick has obtained a college degree, has become a best-selling author, an in-demand motivational speaker who encourages millions of people each year, he started his own ministry, married a lovely young woman, and had his first child. That's not bad for a man around 30 years old (with no limbs!).

Nick is quickly becoming a worldwide phenomenon, and if you ever get the chance, I'd highly recommend you watch some of his videos on YouTube. Nick oozes inspiration and motivation, and after watching his videos, you'll feel as if you have no more excuses for delaying your life or living in defeat (regardless of your "perceived setbacks"). You'll want to get up and achieve something great with your life—hives or no hives.

Conclusion: Get Positive and Stay Motivated

The purpose of this chapter was to offer you a few tips on staying positive and motivated. I'm no stranger to defeat—I've wasted a great many years struggling against feelings of insignificance, worthlessness, and self-pity.

The good news, however, is that you are worth something. There is a purpose for your life, but you have to make the decision to stand up and embrace your destiny. You can play the pity-party game as I did, and you'd have a good enough reason to do so (obnoxious hives).

However, why should you do that? Why live life in a miserable way? Why should you let your hives dictate your happiness, your dreams, and your goals? I was a fool for letting my circumstances control my happiness for so long—don't make the same stupid mistake I did.

Regardless of what's happening in your life, there is hope for tomorrow. I don't care how negative, depressing, or bleak life seems—it can get better in an instant. You may be living in the slums today and in a mansion tomorrow. You can be riddled with cancer and hives today and be healthy tomorrow.

Get up, fight the good fight, hold your head high, and don't give in to life's troubles. You can be a conqueror. You can achieve great things. A better tomorrow awaits you—so embrace each day as if it may be the day your life changes.

Chapter 11: A Few Words for Loved Ones

One of the struggles I faced while suffering with cholinergic urticaria was trying to make my friends, family members, and wife understand what I was going through. It was also challenging trying to make them understand the name of the disorder I had—"You have cholinerg-a-what?"

Therefore, I wanted to write a brief chapter offering some advice and insights to family members. My goal with this chapter is to help them better understand what you're going through and offer them ways to give you the support you'll need during your journey with this disorder.

If you have some friends or family members who are having trouble understanding your pain (literally), then perhaps you can let them read this chapter. Ideally, I recommend they read the entire book.

Understanding a Loved One Suffering with Cholinergic Urticaria

If you're reading this right now, you probably have a loved one suffering with this disorder. Perhaps it's a child, spouse, friend, sibling, or even a parent. If so, you may be wondering why they are suddenly having fits of itching and scratching. In fact, you may have noticed some of their symptoms (or seemingly odd behavior), including:

-Developing small pinpoint hives when they become hot
-Flushing (redness that forms on the skin's surface)
-Wheals (raised areas of the skin)
-Reduced sweating
-Feeling as if they are being "stung" by tiny bees or ants
-Avoiding physical activity or heat
-Breaking out in a frantic scratching episode
-Feeling bouts of frustrating and even depression

All of this can be very frustrating for both of you. Therefore, I'll briefly cover the basics about this disorder.

What Is Cholinergic Urticaria?

Cholinergic urticaria is one of the subtypes of physical urticaria, although some classify it as an "other urticaria type." It is characterized by a hypersensitive response in the skin following an increase in body temperature, especially when the body's temperature increases enough to illicit a sweat response.

To put it another way, cholinergic urticaria is a type of hives that erupts on the skin when a person suffering with the disorder experiences a sudden increase in body temperature.

Your loved one will find it difficult to be in hot rooms, be physically active, and so forth. He or she may have reduced sweating ability, and rather than sweating, he or she will likely break out in an intense "prickly, itchy, stinging feeling."

Describing what this disorder feels like is very difficult, simply because it is impossible to imagine what it feels like unless you've actually felt it. It itches—but itching is only the tip of the iceberg. It also stings, but stinging comes in waves. It's kind of like having a severe case of poison ivy while also being attacked by fire ants.

This disorder can last for years, even decades. There is no "cure," but there are many ways to treat or manage it (see the chapter on treatments), and sometimes it even goes away on its own spontaneously.

In my own case, my hives went away when I eliminated troublesome foods from my diet, along with a few other things (see the chapter "How I Cured My Cholinergic Urticaria"). However, each person may have a different cause, and diet modifications may not help everyone.

154

What Your Loved One is Feeling

Once your loved one realizes that he or she has cholinergic urticaria, a new onslaught of emotions may begin to affect him or her.

Frustration/Aggravation

It is quite normal for your loved one to feel a sense of frustration or aggravation. It soon becomes a challenge to do normal activity—exercising, walking on a hot day, etc.—without feeling the intense itching and stinging associated with this condition.

There have been many days in which I simply "gave up" and stopped trying to do whatever it was I was trying to do. I can remember trying to change the oil in my car one day, but the heat of the day kept making me break out in the prickly feeling.

I'd pause for a few minutes, and then I'd try to resume the maintenance. After doing this several times, I eventually just stopped. Frustrated, I decided I'd just mess with my car another day.

This can happen in many different ways and in many situations. You're going to have to accept the fact that your loved one has a new challenge in life. They can't do the things they used to do—at least, not without experiencing a horrible sensation on their skin.

Depression

In addition to the frustration your loved may feel from the constant pain of hives, he or she may also experience bouts of depression. This can range from a few minutes of feeling "down" immediately following a hives reaction, to an extended period of bitterness, negativity, and hopelessness.

While I never sought treatment (or a diagnosis) for my depression, I did often go through bouts of it. I often felt a sense of hopelessness, and I often wallowed in my own sense of negativity and self-pity.

Other people suffering with cholinergic urticaria have expressed similar experiences on the cholinergicurticaria.net forum. One person even posted about their having contemplated suicide.

While not every person suffering with this disorder will go through this, your loved one may experience bouts of depression. It is important that you learn to be there for them, and in the event they ever indicate thoughts of suicide, you need to help them get the proper support.

How to Support Your Loved One

Although my wife didn't always understand what I was going through (and even felt frustrated due to her inability to help my condition), she did her best to be there for me during the hard times. Moreover, although you may not know exactly what your loved one is going through, it is important that you be there for them.

Here are some general tips for how you can support your loved one through their health trials:

-Don't suggest it's "all in their heads." While some illnesses may be psychosomatic (meaning, "imagined"), this one is not. This is a real type of hives. Real histamine leaks into the skin, and a real reaction occurs. The stinging is real, and it isn't fun. Telling someone that it is "all in their head" is not only annoying, it's also heartless.

I actually had some people suggest it was all in my head. I always wanted to go over, slap them through the face, and then ask, "Did that hurt?" When they replied, "Yes," then I dreamed of saying, "Hmm, it must just be 'all in your head.'"

156

-Don't take your loved one to some medical quack. While I'm all for natural remedies, cholinergic urticaria is a real hives condition, and there are tons of "quack" cures out there for hives. Don't drag your loved one all over creation and have them take every quack cure under the sun.

Also, don't spend all day Googling cures and then spend a small fortune on them. There are tons of websites out there offering a magical cream, spray, or pill. These cures will not only be ineffective, but they will leave you poorer (and even more frustrated).

Stick with mainstream treatments and real medical doctors. I'd recommend your loved one see a dermatologist or allergist, as they will likely offer the best knowledge about this condition. Help your loved one take the information they learn from this book (and website), and talk to a doctor about what may be safe for him or her to try.

For a guide to common treatments and my experimentation with them, please read the "Cholinergic Urticaria Treatments" chapter. You can also read other's experiences on the cholinergicurticaria.net website.

-Let your loved one "vent." It can be hard dealing with this hives disorder, especially in severe cases. Sometimes your loved one may need to vent their frustrations to you. Even if you can't help them, listening alone can sometimes alleviate stress.

I'd often unload my frustrations on my wife in one big "vent-fest," and she'd sit and listen to me. She rarely said anything that made me feel better, but I noticed that sharing my feelings alone helped tremendously.

If your loved one has never talked about their hives, perhaps you should ask them to share their feelings. Ask them how it affects them, or how they're coping with it.

You may also want to encourage them to stop by the website, cholinergicurticaria.net/hives/forum/, and share their feelings or leave a few comments to help support others who have shared their experiences.

-Be positive and offer encouragement. You need to always be positive and try to encourage your loved one.

Remind them that there are many different treatment options and that this disorder will likely go away one day. Remind them that other people go through what they're going through and that they aren't alone.

If your loved one tells you that they had a hard day, listen to their troubles. Then compliment them on how well they've adapted to the condition so far.

-Learn their hives triggers and limits, and respect them. One of the best things you can do to show support for your loved one is to identify what it is that commonly creates a hives reaction in them. Find out what his or her limits are in normal day-to-day activity, and then respect those limits.

For example, if playing basketball causes your loved one to break out in hives, don't ask them to play every day; it's obnoxious. Asking someone with severe cholinergic urticaria to do a physical activity is like inviting a blind man to the movies, or a person with no legs to go walking. They just aren't going to be able to do most physical activities until they get their hives under control.

It's hard (if not impossible) for people with cholinergic urticaria to do these activities without experiencing pain and trauma, especially if their hives are severe. (As a side note, if you have a child in school, you may want to get a doctor's note to excuse them from gym class).

If your loved one breaks out when he or she eats spicy foods, don't ask them if they want hot sauce on their food, and don't invite them to a spicy restaurant. Alternatively, if your loved one is a spouse, you need to understand that they may not be able to be intimate with you like they once did. Some things may have to change during physical intimacy to accommodate his or her hives.

The fact that my loved ones often forgot about my "triggers" was a great source of frustration for me. Even after telling them that I can't do "X" activity, or that I can't eat "X" foods, they continued to offer or invite me. I just got to a point where I really began to get aggravated with them.

If you want to garner a lot of respect from your loved one whom is suffering with hives, you'll go a long way if you simply listen to them and respect what they tell you. Memorize what causes their triggers, and help them avoid those situations. Don't entice them to join you in some activity that will cause a hives attack.

My wife was great about this when I was suffering. For example, if I was in a grocery store checking out with her in line and she noticed I suddenly started scratching myself, she'd say, "You can go on to the car and I'll finish checking out."

We had this down so well that I could often just scratch my forehead, and she'd know an attack was coming. I also had another way of doing this. I could say, "I'm going to go to the car, okay?" and she'd know exactly what I was doing.

By doing that, it allowed me to leave the grocery store discreetly while also avoiding a dreadful hives attack. I'd then usually get in the car, crank up the air conditioner, and scratch myself silly until my hives subsided.

We also had to modify our routines quite a bit. I'd mow in the morning so I could avoid the mid-day heat. When my hives were worst, my wife would even take over and mow for me, which made me feel loved but also bad for having to let her do it.

Conclusion

In summary, pay attention to what triggers your loved one's hives. Try your best to help him or her avoid those activities. Be his or her support partner, and help them in every way you can.

Offer your loved one a shoulder to cry on. Be their advocate when it comes to school, work, etc. Help arrange your lifestyle so that they can avoid unnecessary hives attacks—at least until they get their hives under control.

If you do that, I guarantee they'll notice—and he or she will appreciate it more than you'll ever know.

Chapter 12: Thirty Days and 18 Steps to Improve Cholinergic Urticaria

If you're struggling with cholinergic urticaria symptoms, you may feel desperate. In fact, the number one question most people ask on the CholinergicUrticaria.net forum is this: "How can I make my hives better?"

I know how hard it can be living with this disorder, so I've put together a "Thirty days and 18 Steps to Improve Cholinergic Urticaria" action plan of what I would suggest to anyone who asked me for my advice on improving their hives.

Think of this plan as something I would say if a friend came up to me and asked for my advice on how he or she could make their hives better. I developed this plan so that you can get into a mode of being proactive about your hives and (hopefully) reduce or eliminate your symptoms. You should be able to complete it in about one month (or 4-6 weeks).

I based this "challenge" on my own success in controlling my symptoms, and while it may not work for everyone, I sincerely pray it works for you. The idea is to reduce all sources of inflammation (or allergic responses) in your body that could be responsible for causing or inflaming your hives. It will also help you eliminate major food allergies, environmental allergies, and so forth.

I'll also warn you: Some of the things on this list will take a tremendous amount of self-will and discipline. If you fall short, pick yourself back up and try again. I've failed myself at times, and I've struggled just like you.

It also may cost a minor amount of money to do this challenge, but it shouldn't take much money at all. You can always buy things over time or clip coupons. If you can't afford some of the things, you don't have to buy them. However, I would at least try the diet portion of the challenge.

Lastly, I acknowledge that I am not a doctor or expert. By doing this challenge, you assume full responsibility for any negative or dangerous consequences that may result from trying it. You agree not to hold me liable for any damages, health problems, or other problems that may arise from trying this challenge (or any other material in this book).

Are you ready for the "Thirty day, 18-step" challenge? Let's begin.

Step 1: Talk to a Doctor

Safety is important. Some of the treatments, diets, or ideas mentioned in this book could be dangerous or even fatal for you if you don't take steps to ensure they're safe for you personally. For example, if you tried an antihistamine while nursing, it could cause harm to your baby. Therefore, this first day involves taking the proper safety precautions by making an appointment with a doctor.

You should discuss the diet, treatment options, this "challenge," and anything else you plan to try from this book in an attempt to make your hives better. **DO NOT** try any suggestions from this book (or cholinergicurticaria.net website) before getting the approval from a qualified medical doctor. If you do not have health insurance or a primary doctor, you may be able to visit a walk-in clinic or something similar.

Moreover, it would be a great time to get a general check-up to rule out any other diseases or disorders that may be causing your hives.

Step 2: Start a Journal

You'll need a way to gauge your progress, so I highly recommend you keep a journal. It doesn't have to be anything fancy; a spiral notebook will do.

Write down your diet each day, and make a note about the severity of your hives. Also, make a note of any medications you try, reactions you have, and so forth. You can also use your journal to make a list of questions to ask your doctor, or to make notes of what your doctor said during the visit.

The idea of using a journal is to make a log related to your hives, diet, and activities each day. This will help you locate any patterns. For example, if you notice a severe hives attack, you can look back at your log and see what you've eaten the previous day, or you can see if something else may have led to the stronger reaction.

Be sure to write the date, your diet, how your hives were that day, and any other important details.

Step 3: Change Your Diet

Since diet made the biggest impact for me, and since it will take the longest to see results from changing your diet, it makes sense to start this early. I've talked at great length in the "Cholinergic Urticaria and Diet" chapter about my own diet experimentation.

You can try any elimination diet that your doctor approves, but since my diet works for me, you may want to use it. The only foods I eat on my "strict' diet are turkey, broccoli, sweet potatoes, white rice with real maple syrup, bananas, strawberries, and blueberries. I eat as often as necessary to feel full, but that's all I eat.

Reminder: Ask your doctor if this diet will be safe for you for at least one month.

If you have a food allergy to any of those foods, or any other health issues (such as diabetes), you can supplement the troublesome food for something else that has a low allergic potential.

In addition, it isn't abnormal to have intense cravings for foods—particularly foods you may have an allergy to. When I started the diet, I often had intense food cravings for food that causes significant allergic responses in my body.

Step 4: Stop All Recreational Drugs or Supplements

If you take any recreational drugs, stop taking them. This includes things like marijuana, alcohol, cigarettes, cocaine, and anything else. This will rule out the potential of them causing an increased allergic response.

In addition, if you are taking over-the-counter supplements such as protein powder, stop taking them for the challenge as well.

Do not stop taking any drugs or supplements that your doctor has advised you to take. If you are unsure, check with your doctor before discontinuing use.

Again, the idea here is to remove any unnecessary sources of allergens. Alcohol alone can make cholinergic urticaria symptoms worse the next day.

Step 5: Consider Taking a Probiotic and Multivitamin

Since probiotics can affect the immune system, and since I've noticed a definite decrease in allergic response while taking them, I'd recommend trying them. Digestive Advantage, Align, and Culturelle are some of the three most highly recommended brands.

I also take a daily multivitamin (Centrum). This ensures I receive all of the vitamins and minerals I need since my diet isn't robust. The only advice I'd give about multivitamins is to take them with a large meal. If you don't, they can cause a slight stomach bloat/upset for a little while.

As always, talk to a doctor before trying either of the above supplements.

Taking a multivitamin can help ensure that you don't develop any vitamin deficiencies. Of course, you can always have your doctor run some tests to rule out any pre-existing deficiencies.

Step 6: Eliminate Lotions, Creams, Perfumes, and Cleansers

There's always a possibility that lotion or cleansers you use could be adding to inflaming your hives symptoms. If you put anything on your body, consider stopping it and replacing it with a hypoallergenic brand. Again, if this is something a doctor has prescribed, follow your doctor's orders.

Remember, after the challenge you can always reintroduce them.

Step 7: Eliminate Soaps, Detergents, and Deodorant

It's also a good idea to eliminate any body wash, soaps, detergents, etc. that will come into contact with your skin. Any added chemical could cause a reaction or increase in inflammation. Instead, switch to hypoallergenic soaps, detergents, etc.

I use Dove Sensitive Skin soap, Arm and Hammer aluminum-free deodorant, and All Free Clear detergent.

Step 8: Eliminate Environmental Allergens

Try to change the filters in your furnace/central air conditioner often, and consider buying a hypoallergenic filter. These usually cost a bit more, but they can help cut down on unnecessary allergens circulating in your home.

Also, use good home cleaning habits to help reduce dust build-up. If you have pets, try to avoid them as much as possible during this challenge. While I love animals, they shed pet dander and roll around in many allergens outside—these things could make your hives worse.

Step 9: Make Your Bed Allergy-free

Consider buying an allergy-free covering for your bedding. This can help cut down on pet dander, dust mites, and so forth. Be sure to wash your sheets at least once a week, preferably twice a week during this challenge. Use a good hypoallergenic detergent as I mentioned previously.

Step 10: Use a High Quality Lotion

While I told you previously to avoid most lotions, I do advise using lotions that have a high rating for skin conditions such as eczema or dermatitis. One lotion that I found that works well is Eucerin Calming Crème. I put it on my skin once per day during the summer, and twice per day during the winter months.

Dermatologists often rate this lotion highly, and it will help soothe, protect, and heal any dry skin, which can aggravate your hives.

Step 11: Use a Humidifier

If you live in a dry climate, or experience low humidity during winter months, I'd highly recommend investing in a small humidifier. Low humidity sucks the oils and moisture from your skin, leaving it dry. This dryness can aggravate cholinergic urticaria, making symptoms worse.

I use a small humidifier made by a "Crane." It doesn't use a filter, and has adjustable settings. I bought it on Amazon.com for around $50. Other models are cheaper, but they may use a filter.

Humidifiers will help keep your skin moisturized. They can also help keep your nasal passages moist.

Step 12: Buy a Showerhead Filter

Tap water can contain many chemicals that can irritate and dry the skin. Chlorine, copper, and other chemicals are just a few that may be in your water supply. To combat this, you can consider purchasing a showerhead filter.

166

I bought a Culligan shower filter for around $15-20, and I only replace the filter cartridge about once or twice a year. It was super easy to install, and I did it within probably 10 minutes. You don't even need any tools other than perhaps pliers to tighten it up snugly. You can also find them at most major home improvement stores.

This can help keep your skin from drying out excessively, which can make your hives symptoms worse.

Step 13: Get Some Motivation and Inspiration

Now is a good time to stop and evaluate your mental state. How are you feeling? Are you feeling overwhelmed? Stressed? Discouraged?

It's easy to feel a mix of emotions as you try this challenge, and I even felt them myself. However, try to find some motivation. Read over the "Getting Motivated and Staying Positive" chapter again if necessary, and apply those tips to your life.

You can get your hives to a place where you can better manage them. Don't lose hope, and don't give up. This takes time because your body doesn't heal overnight. Just as it takes many days for a cut to heal on your skin, it also takes many days for inflammation to decrease.

Step 14: Get an EpiPen

Since this challenge will include exercise, it's important to talk to a doctor about an EpiPen. This device can help in the case of anaphylactic shock. It's relatively rare for this to happen to people with cholinergic urticaria, but it's always possible. Try to get one, and always have it handy while exercising.

Step 15: Obtain Cardio Exercise Equipment

Before you begin an exercise program, I highly recommend you obtain some basic equipment. If you prefer to run outdoors, have a membership at a local gyp, or already own equipment, that's fine. Owning your own exercise equipment will make it much easier to exercise, and you won't have to worry about the added aggravation or expense of dealing with a gym membership.

I recommend a stationary bike or elliptical for cardio, although you can use any method or machine you feel comfortable using.

Step 16: Begin Cardio Exercise

Assuming your doctor has approved your exercise regimen, it's time to begin with cardio exercise. My advice is to follow the same strategy I used in the "Cholinergic Urticaria and Exercise" chapter. I'd stop at the first sign of a serious attack, and then I'd cool off. Once my hives subsided, I'd begin again.

Try to get at least 20-30 minutes of cardio each day and at least 3-5 days of exercise per week. Be sure to stretch or warm-up to prevent injury. In addition, it is always a great idea to have your EpiPen and an exercise partner nearby—just in case you ever have a severe attack.

Note: I do not recommend exercise for those who have experienced anaphylactic shock, have anhidrosis or severe hypohidrosis (reduced or lack of sweating function), people with other health problems that may prevent exercise, or those with abnormally severe cholinergic urticaria. If your doctor recommends not exercising, please follow your doctor's advice.

Step 17: If You're Overweight, Start Losing Weight

Carrying around excess fat can increase inflammation and cause other health risks. If you're overweight, I'd advise you to talk with your doctor and put together a plan to get to a healthy weight. If you're already a healthy weight, then strive to stay healthy.

Most experts agree that the best way to lose weight is slowly over time via exercise and proper diet. Don't try extreme diets, and don't starve yourself, as this often backfires. However, by cutting just 500 calories per day, you can lose roughly one pound per week. That may not sound like much, but even 10 pounds can make a huge difference in your health and weight.

Granted, the diet and exercise program recommended in this book may help you lose weight. Ultimately, it will depend on how many calories you consume and how many you burn while exercising. I'd recommend you use a free calorie calculator on the Internet to determine the amount of calories you need to consume to lose one pound per week, and ask your doctor what your ideal weight should be. Consult a nutritional or fitness expert for more personalized suggestions on losing weight.

Step 18: Consider Adding Weights to Your Routine

After doing cardio for at least two weeks, you may want to consider adding a few simple weights for some strength training. You don't need anything fancy—a few dumbbells will do. You'd be amazed at the number of exercises you can do with just two or three dumbbells of different weight.

I've given some sample exercise routines in the exercise chapter, and you can find plenty of sample routines online. It's very important to stretch, use proper form, and have a spotter when doing exercises with weight. If you are unsure how to perform the exercises, consult with a fitness trainer.

How Long Should You Try the Steps?

Once I did everything mentioned above (diet, exercise, etc.), it took about 4-6 weeks for my cholinergic urticaria symptoms to decrease to the point where I could sweat and no longer break out. The first indicator that my hives were improving was when I broke through and sweat for the first time in a long time.

I know it may be hard doing the diet and exercise, but if your doctor agrees that it's safe for you, I'd highly recommend you do it for 4-6 weeks to see if it helps. If it does help, at least you'll know how to manage your hives in a new way. If it doesn't help, at least you'll know, and you can return to your old diet and products.

This "challenge" above has been a lifesaver for me. It has completely changed my life. Whether it will help you, I cannot say. I pray it does help you.

What if the Regimen Doesn't Work for You?

If you try all of the steps above and get no relief from your hives, then there is still hope for you. Don't get frustrated. Remember that this probably won't last forever, and that many people have been where you are now (including me).

My advice would be to carefully read over the "Cholinergic Urticaria Treatments" chapter, and start with the safest treatment options available. Work with a doctor to try different approaches until your hives get better. Treatments like antihistamines may provide some relief with minimal side effects. Other treatments are available to help you cope with symptoms.

Life can be hard when you have cholinergic urticaria, but it's not impossible. Many sufferers have found ways to manage their hives, and I know that in time you will as well. You can beat this condition.

Final Words

Cholinergic urticaria nearly destroyed my life. It's also been an odd source of great blessings. Through all of my struggles, I've learned a lot. I've learned to be more positive and to count my blessings. I've learned that life can change in an instant. I've learned that our health is fragile—we should cherish and protect it.

When I wrote this book, my main goal was to do three things: Educate people about cholinergic urticaria, share my own experiences and "cure," and provide a strategy so that people can work with their doctors to reduce their symptoms. I've tried my very best to do those three things, and I pray that you've found this book useful.

This book contains everything I have to say on this subject. It sums up my entire knowledge and experience with this condition, and I've tried to make it as detailed and comprehensive as possible in an effort to help others.

If this book has helped you, please help spread the word so that others may get some benefit as well. Consider letting others know on social media, your blog, or whatever else.

Moreover, if you'd like to share your story or experience, or ask questions to a community of people suffering with cholinergic urticaria, I'd like to invite you to do so here: http://www.cholinergicurticaria.net/hives/forum/.

If you do post a question, I ask that you consider answering at least one other person's question. This way, it doesn't become a forum with many questions and no answers. A give-take approach works well in online communities, and the forum would be great if everyone answered one question for each question asked.

Moreover, I rarely participate in the forum these days, and I've mostly created it for the community of people suffering to share and ask questions. However, I do try to respond to questions that I haven't already addressed in this book (or website) when I have time.

You can also subscribe to posts and comments if you'd like to keep up with any new information posted on the website or forum.

I pray that this book has helped you in some way, and I pray your hives get better soon. Hang in there. You will beat this thing.

Love,

Ben (Hivesguy)

74505786R00096

Made in the USA
Columbia, SC
04 August 2017